GENETIC EPIDEMIOLOGY AND MOLECULAR GENETIC ANALYSIS

G. NANDHINI

CONTENTS

LIST OF ABBREVIATIONS

LIST OF TABLES

LIST OF FIGURES

1. INTRODUCTION	1-3
2. REVIEW OF LITERATURE	4-33
3. METHODOLOGY	34-50
4. RESULTS	51-96
5. DISCUSSION	97-111
6. SUMMARY AND CONCLUSION	112-117

LIST OF ABBREVIATIONS

Abbreviation		Term description
ACC	-	Anterior Cingulate Cortex
ADARB2	-	Adenosine Deaminase RNA Specific B2 (Inactive)
ADHD	-	Attention deficit hyperactive disorder
ANKK1	-	Ankyrin repeat and kinase domain containing 1 gene
AP4E1	-	Adaptor Protein complex 4 Epsilon subunit 1
ARNT2	-	Aryl Hydrocarbon Receptor Nuclear Translocator 2
ASD	-	Autism Spectrum disorder
BGTC	-	Basal Ganglia Thalamo-cortical loop
CNS	-	Central Nervous system
CNTNAP2	-	Contactin Associated Protein Like 2
CTNNA3	-	Catenin Alpha 3
CWS	-	Children With Stuttering
DRD2	-	Dopamine receptor D2 gene
ECM	-	Extra cellular matrix
ES	-	Exome sequencing
EYA2	-	Eyes absent
FADS2	-	Fatty acid desaturase
FMN1	-	Formin 1
fNIRS	-	Functional Near Infrared Spectroscopy
FOXP2	-	Forkhead box protein P2
GAGs	-	Glycosaminoglycans
GIF	-	Genealogical index of families
GMV	-	Grey Matter Volume

GNPTAB	-	GlcNAc-1-phosphotransferase alpha and beta subunits
GNPTG	-	gamma subunit of GlcNAc-1-phosphotransferase enzyme
IFG	-	Inferior Frontal Gyrus
LOD	-	Logarithm of Odds
MRI	-	Magnetic resonance imaging
NAGPA	-	N-acetylglucosamine-1-phosphodiester alpha-N acetyl glucosaminidase
NLRP11	-	NOD like receptor protein 11
NMJ	-	Neuromuscular junction
OASES	-	Overall Assessment of the Speaker's Experience of Stuttering
OMIM	-	Online Mendelian Inheritance in Man
PCSK5	-	Proprotein Convertase Subtilisin/Kexin Type 5
PFC	-	Probability of familial clustering
PLXNA4	-	Plexin A4
PNS	-	Peripheral Nervous System
SLC24A3	-	Solute Carrier Family 24 Member 3
SLC6A3	-	Solute Carrier Family 6 Member 3
SMA	-	Supplementary Motor Area
SNS	-	Sympathetic nervous system
STG	-	Superior-Temporal Gyrus
Taq	-	*Thermus aquaticus*
TISA	-	The Indian stammering association
UCE	-	Uncovering enzyme
VBM	-	Voxel-based morphometry
VUS	-	Variant with unknown significance

LIST OF TABLES

Table 1:	Distribution of different mutations in *GNPTAB, GNPTG & NAGPA* genes implicated in stuttering
Table 2:	Compilation of genetic studies in numerous multiplex families worldwide (2002- 2017)
Table 3:	Overview of mutations in stuttering vs. mucolipidosis
Table 4:	Primer pairs of *GNPTAB, GNPTG & NAGPA* used for PCR and DNA sequencing
Table 5:	Real time nucleotide primer sequences of target (*GNPTAB, GNPTG, NAGPA*) and endogenous (β-actin) genes
Table 6:	Comparison of sex ratio (familial Vs sporadic) among person with stuttering
Table 7:	Frequency distribution of children with stuttering in relation to age and sex ratios
Table 8:	Frequency of stuttering among the relatives of male and female probands
Table 9:	Manner of onset among stuttering probands
Table 10:	Frequency of stuttering among first-, second- and third-degree relatives of probands with a positive family history
Table 11:	Distribution of parental consanguinity among sporadic and familial stuttering probands
Table 12:	Frequency of parental consanguinity and the coefficient of inbreeding among stuttering probands
Table 13:	Frequency of parental consanguinity in stuttering probands by religion
Table 14:	Stress factors studied among stuttering probands
Table 15:	Distribution of severity of stuttering among the probands
Table 16:	Risk factors for severity of stuttering for school da
Table 17:	Risk factors for severity of stuttering for hospital data
Table 18:	Familial Aggregation indices of both school and hospital data
Table 19:	Allele frequencies of the 12 gene variants observed in *GNPTAB, GNPTG* and *NAGPA* genes among the 64 stuttering probands and comparison with gnomAD database

Table 20:	Pathogenicity prediction of the variants observed in three stuttering genes using various bioinformatics tools
Table 21:	Lysosomal enzyme study in the plasma of a stuttering family
Table 22:	Variant profile of the probands in the three putative genes for stuttering
Table 23:	Segregation pattern and genotype-phenotype correlation of likely pathogenic variants identified in the three putative genes for stuttering among the 64 probands screened
Table 24:	Compilation of the variants common in parent offspring pair of STU 66 family correlating to speech language disorders that includes 15 novel variants observed along with the bioinformatic predictions for pathogenicity
Table 25:	Characterization of the stuttering phenotype and other associated findings among 24 individuals examined in the STU 65 family
Table 26:	Compilation of the variants common in sib pair of STU 65 family correlating to speech language disorders that includes 8 novel variants observed along with the bioinformatic predictions for pathogenicity
Table 27:	Manually curated list of candidate* genes identified in putative pathways, that can be directly or indirectly linked to stuttering, in the two families studied
Table 28:	Over-representation analysis results of variants identified in two ES families showing 25 most significant pathways related to stuttering using Reactome database
Table 29:	Tentative list of candidate* genes identified in enrichment pathways, that can be directly or indirectly linked to stuttering, in the two families studied

LIST OF FIGURES

Figure 1: The two pathways utilized in speech production involving auditory cortex or visual cortex

Figure 2: Overview of speech and language disorders

Figure 3: Types of dysfluencies in normal and stuttering individuals

Figure 4: Core, secondary and psychological behaviours observed in stuttering

Figure 5: Membrane bound GlcNAc-1-phosphotransferase complex activation

Figure 6: M6P tagging for transport of lysosomal enzyme

Figure 7: (a) GNPTAB (b) GNPTG gene exonic mutation spectrum so far reported in stuttering. Red colour variants indicates the ones also reported in mucolipidosis

Figure 8: Salem and Chennai city maps showing the location of the schools screened

Figure 9: Flow chart depicting the study design and recruitment of 342 children with stuttering used for epidemiological study in phase I

Figure 10: RNA integrity analysis by agarose gel electrophoresis. The 28S and 18S rRNA bands are indicated. The lanes L1-4 represents four samples and L5-8 are duplicates with different dilution

Figure 11: Melt curve plot from qPCR of (A) *GNPTAB* (B) *GNPTG* (C) *NAGPA* (D) All three genes along with β-actin control gene

Figure 12: Schematic representation of the exome sequencing workflow

Figure 13: Bioinformatics analysis pipeline adapted from MedGenome's protocol

Figure 14: An Upset plot of identified variants in this study across three genes implicated in stuttering to show combination of variants among probands. For each variant that is a part of intersection, a black filled circle is shown in the matrix and for the variant that is not part of intersection, a light gray circle is placed. The number of probands bearing the set of variants (column-based relationships) is emphasized by vertical black line connecting the top most and bottom most black circle. The bar chart on top and left of the matrix gives the size of intersections and sets respectively.

Figure 15: Partial chromatograms of the Glu1200Lys mutation (*GNPTAB*) segregating in a family with stuttering

Figure 16: Partial chromatogram of c.802A>C (Ile268Leu) variation in *GNPTG* gene

Figure 17: The relative levels of *GNPTG*, *GNPTAB*, and *NAGPA* mRNA expression were determined in WBC from blood sample of stuttering patients by real-time PCR normalized to β-actin expression. Data indicates ΔCt values ±SD

Figure 18: Partial chromatogram of c.131G>C (Arg44Pro) mutation in *NAGPA* gene

Figure 19a: MAFFT alignment of native and mutated secondary structure of GNPTAB protein using the Geneious Pro version 6.1.2 identified the loss of helix and addition of turn at the site of mutation.

Figure 19b: MAFFT alignment of native and mutated secondary structure of GNPTG protein using the Geneious Pro version 6.1.2 showing no change in the secondary structure

Figure 20: Five generation pedigree of stuttering family STU 66

Figure 21: Venn diagram showing the variants shared among the four individuals in the STU 66 family (15 combinations)

Figure 22: Bioinformatic-analysis pipeline applied to exome sequence data of a

STU 66 family with stuttering

Figure 23: Six generational pedigree of a stuttering family STU 65

Figure 24: Venn diagram showing the variants shared between the affected sib pair in the STU 65 family

Figure 25: Bioinformatic-analysis pipeline applied to exome sequence data of a STU 65 family with stuttering

Figure 26: Venn diagram showing the genes shared between two stuttering multiplex families

Figure 27: Flow chart depicting exome analysis of two multiplex stuttering families

CHAPTER 1

INTRODUCTION

Speech is a special gift to a human being resulting in the robust means of vocal communication that is unique to him among the extant species. Modern humans' speech and cognitive capabilities are due to **species-specific anatomy** and **neural mechanisms**. In humans, there are two sections in the vocal tracts —a "horizontal" section in the oral cavity (mouth and oropharynx) and a "vertical" section in the throat (pharynx). These two sections form a right angle and are roughly equivalent in length— in a 1:1 proportion, in contrast to primates with disproportionately long horizontal section incapacitating them to produce 'quantal' sounds ([i], [u] and [a]) that are important for speech production. Human speech is also believed to have appeared about 50,000 years ago in Paleolithic fossil record but absent in Neanderthals and earlier humans (Lieberman, 2007).

Speech also calls for a brain that can "repeat"—freely rearrange a **limited set of motor gestures to form a potentially unlimited number of words and sentences**. Current findings contest the conventional theory of localizing the neural bases of human speech and language to Broca's and Wernicke's areas. These cortical areas in unison with other neural circuits are linked to the basal ganglia and subcortical structures which are critical in regulating motor control, speech and language production and cognitive processes together with syntax (Lieberman & Mccarthy, 2007).

Speech is a unique motor accomplishment requiring **coordination of multiple organs** and any disturbance in this harmony results in an array of speech disorders. It involves production of sound by controlled movement of coordinated muscles regulated by rate of breathing and brain activity. The speech function can be hampered to cause both receptive and expressive communication disorders. Expressive speech and language disorders include aphasia, lisp, stuttering and cluttering.

This study focuses on **stuttering** which is one such expressive speech disorder of fluency where the smooth flow of speech is interrupted by involuntary disruptions like **repetitions, prolongations, or blocks and other secondary behaviors** such as head jerks, lip tremors and eye blinks. The symptoms often inflate to **psychological behaviors** which leads to lack of confidence during speech in social situations thereby increasing their anxiety levels with anticipation of stuttering. Stuttering arises in children of 2-5 years of age during the development of speech and language but most of the children (80%) recover spontaneously. Males are preferentially affected than females with a male to female ratio of ~5:1, females having a greater chance of recovery (Drayna *et al.*, 1999; Yairi & Ambrose, 1999; 2005). There are multiple layers of difficulty that often manifest in individual's academic, professional and social life resulting in significantly reduced quality of life and they have the tendency to isolate themselves (Ashurst & Wasson, 2011).

In a comprehensive review on the **epidemiology of stuttering**, Yairi and Ambrose (2012) reported more than 40 prevalence studies worldwide. The prevalence rates ranged from 0.3% to 5.6% and the average prevalence over the lifespan may be lower than the commonly cited 1% that was noted in the last century (Yairi & Ambrose, 2012). In India, to date only three studies (Hegarty, 1968; NSSO, 2003; Srinath *et al.*, 2004) have documented the incidence and prevalence of stuttering in an indirect manner (psychiatric and communication disorders).

Every country needs a credible estimate for the prevalence of stuttering to frame its national policy and effectively tackle the disorder in terms of management. In the **present study,** we attempted a targeted approach to scrutinize the **prevalence of stuttering in India by screening school children**.

The underlying cause for stuttering had been contemplated since antiquity and understanding a complex trait like stuttering requires intensive multidisciplinary effort from various fields like genetics, neuroscience, linguistics, psychology, developmental biology and anthropology (Fisher & Marcus, 2006). Current approaches to find the cause of stuttering are predominated by two different research strategies - neuroimaging and genetic studies. Most of **brain imaging** methods have consistently reported structural or functional differences contributing to inefficient communication in stuttering. White matter abnormalities (Chang *et al.*, 2015) and laterality differences (Cykowski *et al.*, 2008) were accounted but it was not possible to know if these differences are the cause or the result of stuttering due to the significant plasticity of brain (Büchel & Watkins, 2010).

Though the biological predisposition for stuttering is not well understood, the **genetic contribution** was strengthened by four decades of research using family pedigrees in the form of familial incidence, aggregation, segregation, twin and adoption studies (Domingues & Drayna, 2017). Mapping genes is the greatest challenge in stuttering as it is a complex disorder where genetic dissection is made difficult due to gene-gene, gene-environment interactions, genetic heterogeneity, gender bias, incomplete penetrance and phenocopies (Oliveira *et al.*, 2012). In order to identify the stuttering causative genes, several linkage studies were performed in numerous multiplex families that identified four genes, *GNPTAB*, *GNPTG*, *NAGPA* and *AP4E1*, whose combined contribution, was estimated to be 20% (Raza et al., 2016). These four genes pointed to a single process, i.e. intracellular trafficking deficits (Domingues & Drayna, 2017) but the biological mechanism that leads to stuttering is yet to be explored.

No such genetic studies on stuttering have been published till date in India and hence in the present study, molecular genetics investigations were initiated. Before undertaking DNA studies, it was ideal to infer the genetic basis of stuttering in terms of incidence in families and familial aggregation with respect to our Indian population. Moreover, the aim of this study was not only to **assess the recurrence of implicated genes** that influence the risk of individuals to stutter (as replicable findings qualify the role of genes) but also to **explore other pathways involved** in disruption of fluent speech by means of exome sequencing in multiplex families. The **present study** would add information in terms of prevalence, to realize whether stuttering aggregates in families among Indian population, replication of candidate genes and information on new genes that contribute to stuttering. It facilitates our understanding of this enigmatic disorder and also enables us to **develop a stuttering database** that includes multiplex families which could be taken up for further, future investigations.

CHAPTER 2

REVIEW OF LITERATURE

Communication is an exchange of thoughts and information with others and **speech** is a form of communication by language that is unique to humans to express their thoughts, ideas and feelings. Speech not only involves the linguistics (articulatory phonetics) but also paralinguistic aspects of vocalization to convey meaning.

2.1 ANATOMY AND PHYSIOLOGY OF SPEECH

Human communication is an extremely complex system that entails control and coordination of intensely interconnected sensorimotor system. It involves a premotor process and mechanical process.

Premotor process

Speech involves **40,000 neuromuscular events per second** that requires the coordination of over 100 muscles (Logan, 2000). All these movements must be coordinated without any fault, for fluent speech. Our speech perceptions are processed by visual cortex and auditory cortex and transferred to Wernicke's area. Hence the messages that we hear or see are decoded in the Wernicke's area and our speech response is linguistically formulated and produced by the Broca area (Figure 1). The Brain's involvement in speech is mostly unconscious and automatic.

Mechanical process

The production of speech involves five systems viz., respiratory, phonatory, resonatory, articulatory and suprasegmental characteristics, that act in integration (Hall & Guyton, 2011). A deep understanding of the structure and function of the organs involved in speech is critical for diagnosing and treating speech disorders.

During speech production, the air from the lungs acts as a source of energy that vibrates the vocal folds. The raw sound produced is filtered in the pharynx and modified by articulators to produce the desired sound. Thus, speech production involves complex interplay of premotor process involving brain and mechanical process involving the five speech systems. Disturbance in this balanced cascade will result in speech disorder.

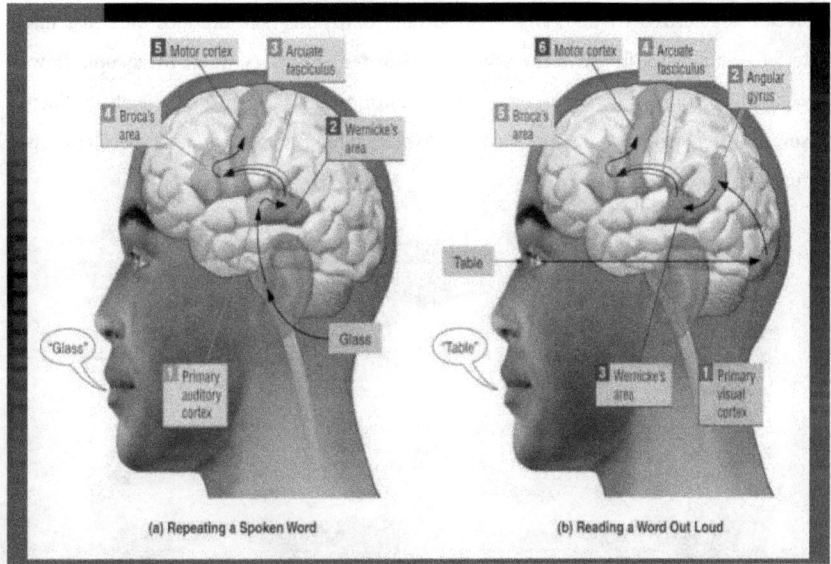

Figure 1: The two pathways utilized in speech production involving auditory cortex or visual cortex (source:https://www.slideshare.net/raghuveer12327/physiology-of-speech-21940437)

2.2 SPEECH DISORDERS

Figure 2 gives an overview of speech and language disorders. They fall under the umbrella of communication disorders and consists of two categories: receptive and expressive.

Receptive language disorders affect one's ability to identify or make sense of sounds and words. **Processing disorder** is one such example in which there is difficulty in understanding and responding. Affected persons often guess what they hear. People with noise filtering disorder are not able to distinguish between surrounding noise and the voice they listen.

Expressive speech and language disorders include aphasia, lisp, stuttering and cluttering. **Aphasia** is the language disorder that affect the production and comprehension of speech and also affects the ability to read and write. **Lisp** is inability to pronounce specific speech sound though they do not have any structural defects. It is the **articulation**

Chapter 2   *Review of literature*

defect characterized by additions or distortion, omissions, substitutions etc., that might interfere with intelligibility. **Stuttering** is a **disorder of fluency** where the smooth flow of speech is interrupted by repetitions, prolongations, or blocks. **Cluttering** is also a fluency disorder that involves excessive breaks due to talking too fast, disorganized speech planning or unsure of what to say.

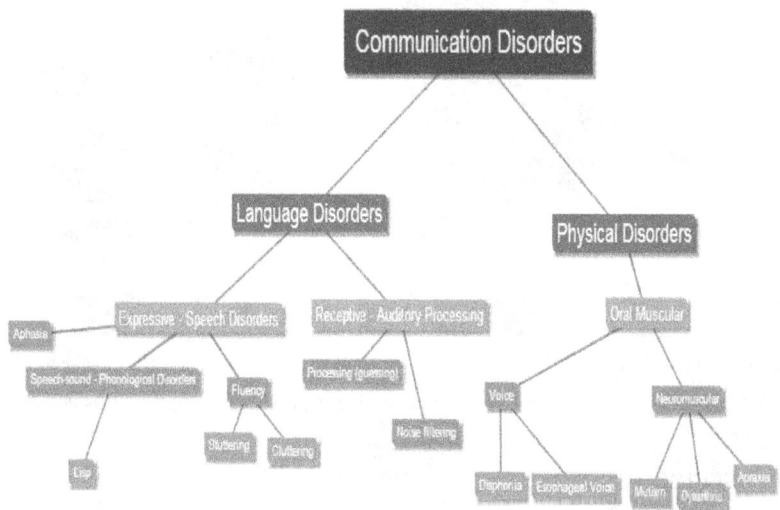

Figure 2: Overview of speech and language disorders (source: https://speechandlanguage disabilities.weebly.com/)

Physical disorders that affect speech are **oral muscular disorders** wherein the muscles that control speech are impaired. It includes **voice disorders** that arise due to swelling of larynx or nerve problems that cause the vocal cords to spasm resulting in esophageal voice and dysphonia. It is characterized by abnormal production of voice, loudness, pitch, altering the voice quality, resonance that is inappropriate for a person's age or sex.

In **neuromuscular disorders** though they have intact speech production center, the muscles and the nerves which control them are affected differentiating from expressive speech disorders. It includes **dysarthria, apraxia and mutism**. Apraxia and dysarthria are motor speech disorders that results in articulation or phonological defects. Apraxia occurs due to problems in planning movement, in absence of any neuromuscular problems. Dysarthria occurs due to problems in execution of movements in the presence of neuromuscular problems. In **mutism** the person is not able to produce speech as they are unable to move their muscles due to damage to the brain or speech muscle. It is an extreme form of aphasia, dysarthria and apraxia (https://speechandlanguagedisabilities. weebly.com/).

2.3 SPEECH FLUENCY

Fluency refers to continuity, rate, smoothness and effort in production of speech. People who are unable to produce fluent speech have speech dysfluency called **stuttering**.

Stuttering Phenotype

Stuttering is a speech disorder characterized by disruption in the fluency, rhythm and timing of speech. The **core behaviors** that manifest are involuntary syllable/part-word *repetitions*, *prolongations* and interruption known as *blocks*. These typical dysfluencies occur at the beginning of sentences, words and sounds (Figure 3). Though Persons With Stuttering (PWS) know what has to be said, but they are unable to initiate the sentence smoothly. Adults who have stuttering develop linguistic escapes such as substitution of words, interjections, revision of sentence, hesitations or tense pauses. Moreover these stuttering events are not static but dynamic and continuous (Prasse & Kikano, 2008).

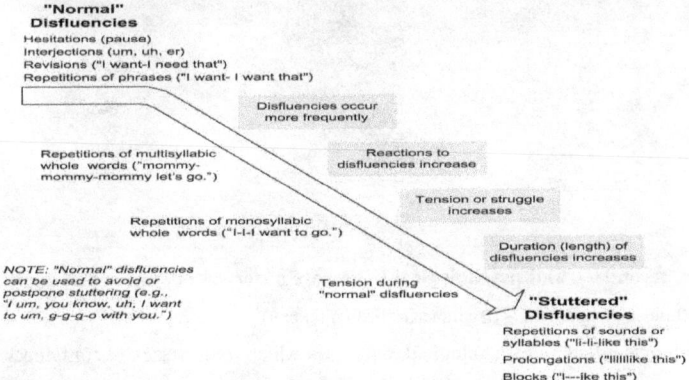

Figure 3: Types of dysfluencies in normal and stuttering individuals
(https://pubs.asha.org)

As the severity progresses dysfluencies are accompanied by **secondary behaviors** depending on the individual. It includes orofacial spastic movements (facial twitching and grimaces, rapid eye blinking, clenching of jaws, jerking movements of the head, raising of upper lip/eyebrow, tremor in lips), movements of hand to the mouth, abnormal breathing, gestures and bodily tensions.

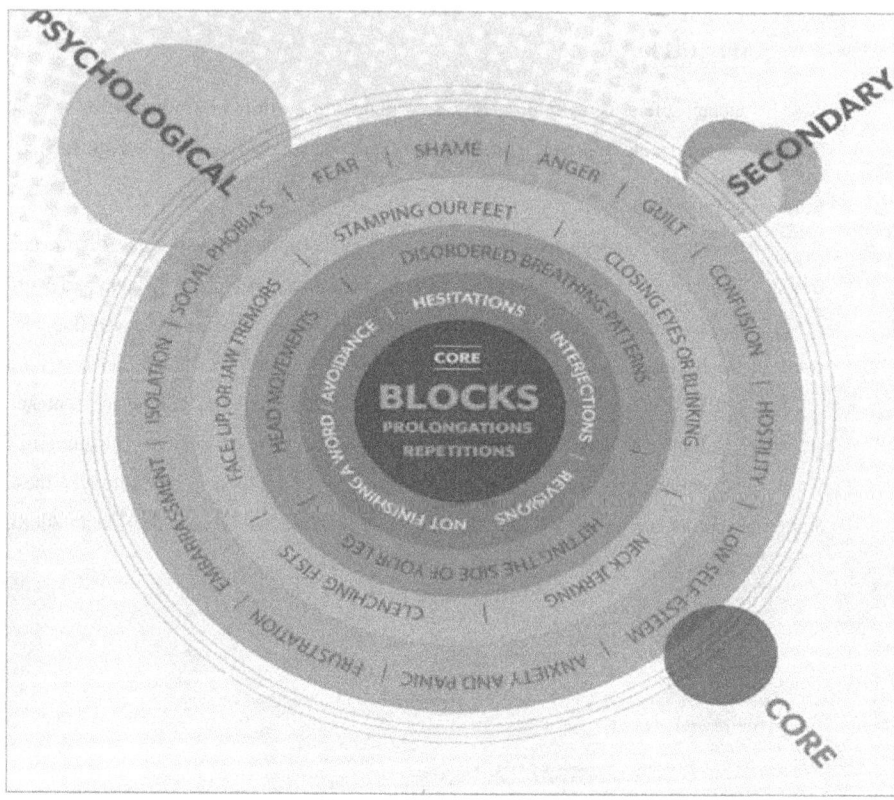

Figure 4: Core, secondary and psychological behaviors observed in stuttering (source: htttps://www.cddft.nhs.uk/media/612541/stammering%20onion.png)

The symptoms inflate to **psychological behaviors** which leads to lack of confidence during speech in social situations thereby increasing their anxiety levels with anticipation of stuttering (Figure 4). Fear of recurrence is mainly due to previous unpleasant speaking experiences. Consequently, they develop embarrassment, shame and feel trapped. In an effort to hide stuttering they build defensive efforts to escape, hide and avoid speech trouble. These personality changes occur in either suppressing their personality or accepting the presence of stuttering. These layers of difficulty often manifest in individuals academic, professional and social life and results in significantly reduced quality of life (Ashurst & Wasson, 2011). PWS are fluent when speaking to themselves, babies, in chorus, singing, paced speech etc., (Kalinowski, & Saltuklaroglu, 2003) but their fluency decreases if planned speech sound is syntactically complex or long (Karniol, 1995).

2.4 CLASSIFICATION OF STUTTERING

a. Based on developmental course - Persistent or Recovery

The typical age of development of stuttering ranges from 30-48 months, the period during which there is rapid speech and language development. Approximately 5-8% of children experience stuttering with a male to female ratio of 1.5:1. About 80% of them *recover* spontaneously (within 18 months) without any aid of therapy, and 20% remain *persistent* (stutter > 36 months) (Månsson, 2000; Gordon, 2002). Hence the prevalence drops to 1% in adults with a male to female ratio of 4:1. The disorder *preferentially affects males* and the remarkable change, in male/female ratio from school age to adult points toward higher rate of recovery among females (Yairi & Ambrose, 2005; 2013).

b. Based on etiology - Developmental, Neurogenic or Psychogenic

Stuttering can be classified as developmental or acquired based on their etiology. **Developmental stuttering** is the most common form with gradual onset. It occurs between 3-8 years of age, the period during which there is extensive speech and language development, hence the term developmental. Preschoolers undergo spontaneous recovery within 4 years. **Acquired stuttering** that arises secondary to brain damage or emotional trauma, are referred to as neurogenic or psychogenic respectively. **Neurogenic stuttering** is rare in occurrence and often lack secondary behaviors. The common neurological diagnosis reported in stuttering were head injury, cortical and subcortical lesions, neurodegenerative disease like Alzheimer and Parkinson, seizures, ADHD, stroke etc., (Ashurst & Wasson, 2011).

Psychogenic stuttering is also a rare form that is characterized by rapid repetition of initial sounds of words. Occurrence is usually due to depression, anxiety, personality disorder, hysteria, drug abuse, etc. Psychogenic stuttering also has overlapping features with neurogenic stuttering but were more frequently associated with struggle behavior and rapid recovery during treatment (Baumgartner & Duffy, 1997).

c. **Based on co-occurrence of stuttering with other disorders - syndromic or non-syndromic**

Stuttering albeit occur by itself without any associated signs or symptoms (**non-syndromic**), also arise as a characteristic feature in various other disorders and syndromes (**syndromic**).

Children Who Stutter (CWS) exhibit co-occurring speech disorders, language disorders and also non-speech language disorders (62.8%). Articulation (33%) and phonology (12%) disorders are highest and voice disorder (2%) is considerably less among co-occurring disorders. Specific Language impairment (SLI) along with stuttering account for 6% indicating the need for language assessment in CWS. Learning disabilities (11%) and attention deficit hyperactive disorders (5.9%) co-occur with stuttering. Another remarkable finding is that males have higher percentage of co-occurrence of speech and non-speech disorders than females but there is no difference for language categories (Blood *et al.*, 2003).

Various genetic syndromes like **Down syndrome, Prader-Willi, Tourette, Fragile X, Turner and Neurofibromatosis type I** have listed stuttering as a primary symptom associated with it. Most extensive review to date by Shprintzen (1997) reports the status of communication disorders in 334 syndromes, mentions the occurrence of stuttering in only a few of them. Syndromes such as Down's, Fragile X, Tourette and Prader-Willi are closely linked with a fluency disorder. In Turner and Neurofibromatosis type I knowledge is only anecdotal due to little data available on frequency and nature of occurrence (Borsel & Tetnowski, 2007).

In Tourette syndrome and Prader-Willi syndrome, in depth analysis of speech behaviors indicate, that the **dysfluency** is not typical of stuttering. In Tourette syndrome the word-medial and word-final **disfluencies** seems to be characteristic disfluency patterns. Word-final disfluencies were observed in Prader-Willi syndrome with absence of secondary behaviors. These disfluency patterns in the two syndromes have the prospective for differential diagnosis; however, Down syndrome and Fragile X have dysfluency patterns similar to developmental stuttering. Hence it is understood that a more in-depth analysis of speech is required for differential diagnosis of **non-fluency** in genetic syndromes. Thus in genetic syndromes the administering of fluency inducing strategies can result in some specific reactions that serve as clues for differential diagnosis of disfluency that is exclusive to this group (Borsel & Tetnowski, 2007).

Stuttering is also considered as a disorder of motor control as it shares a number of characteristics with dystonia, dyspraxia, dysarthria, Tourett's syndrome and Parkinson (Ludlow & Loucks, 2003). Stuttering is also reported in schizophrenia (Nagendrappa *et al.*, 2019), Autism (Alaghband-Rad *et al.*, 2013) and bipolar disorders as side effects to drugs or high anxiety levels.

2.5 EPIDEMIOLOGY OF STUTTERING

Since 2000 six major studies (Månsson, 2000; Felsenfeld *et al.*, 2000; Craig *et al.*, 2002; Månsson, 2005; Dworzynski *et al.*, 2007; Reilly *et al.*, 2009) worldwide reported on the incidence of stuttering as 5-18% that mainly focused on Caucasian populations. On the other hand seven studies during the same time reported on its prevalence since 2000 (Okalidou & Kampanaros, 2001; Craig *et al.*, 2002; van Borsel *et al.*, 2006; McKinnon *et al.*, 2007; Proctor *et al.*, 2008; McLeod & Harrison, 2009; Boyle *et al.*, 2011) in the range between 0.33 to 5.6%. Craig *et al.*, reports both incidence rate (5%) and the average prevalence in adult population as 1% (2002).

In India, to date only three studies have documented the incidence and prevalence of stuttering in an indirect manner, where the prevalence of stuttering was reported from studies on psychiatric and communication disorders. An early pilot survey on the incidence of speech handicaps among Indian school children in New Delhi, from kindergarten to seventh grade, indicated a prevalence of 1.2% for stuttering (Hegarty, 1968). A National survey conducted by the Government of India on various disabilities reported 0.4% prevalence among disabled persons (NSSO, 2003). An epidemiological study of child and adolescent psychiatric disorders reported a prevalence rate of stuttering as 1.5% among 4-16 years-old from urban, slum and rural areas of Bangalore, Karnataka (Srinath et al., 2004). However, the All India Institute of Speech and Hearing (AIISH) found 10% stuttering among children with communication disorders (Subramanian & Prabhu, 2005).

Risk factors for stuttering

The etiology of stuttering is still largely unknown although several risk factors have been reported, including low birth weight (Boulet et al., 2011; McAllister & Collier, 2014), age and manner of onset (Yairi & Ambrose, 2005), gender (Ambrose et al., 1997), severity (Prasse & Kikano, 2008), positive parental stuttering/family history (Kloth et al., 1998), and attitude towards the disorder and treatment (Bothe et al., 2006; Subramanian & Prabhu, 2005). Exploration of these risk factors may help in recognizing stuttering early, thus enabling timely intervention.

Age at onset: The age at onset for developmental stuttering is 2-5 years, whereas the adult-onset type is considered as acquired and may be further sub-classified as neurogenic and psychogenic (Wittke-Thompson *c* 2007). Developmental stuttering mostly affects children, with a gradual onset (Prasse & Kikano, 2008). Age at onset is reported to be associated with persistency (Cox et al., 1984), and Yairi and Ambrose (2005) reported that a trend for persistency is associated with later age at onset. The phenomenon of spontaneous recovery has been extensively discussed in the scientific literature (Bloodstein, 1995).

Sex Ratio: At all ages there is a skewed *sex ratio* with a preponderance of males affected (Drayna & Kang, 2011; Gordon, 2002). The higher chronicity of the disorder among males than females generally has been explained by the fact that the females have a greater tendency for recovery than males (Ambrose et al., 1997).

Severity: Speech assessment establishes the *severity* of dysfluency, which can be classified as normal, mild and severe. In severe cases, stuttering occurs in almost every phrase and it may be accompanied by secondary behaviors such as eye blinking, heard jerks, lip pressing etc., resulting in embarrassment and fear of speaking (Prasse & Kikano, 2008).

Family history: Several studies, including twin and family reports, have demonstrated the involvement of genetic factors in the transmission of susceptibility to stuttering, therefore *family history* is an important risk factor (Domingues & Drayna, 2017). Statistical evidence for both a single major locus and a polygenic component have been advocated in persistent and recovered stuttering (Ambrose *et al.*, 1997).

Consanguinity: *Consanguinity* is the union of individuals genetically related to each other as close or closer than second cousins ($F \geq 0.0156$). Intracommunity marriage is the norm in most regions that favor consanguineous marriages, e.g., within castes in India, and in such circumstances gene flow between communities is highly restricted. Consanguinity has a greater influence on the etiology of complex diseases when rare autosomal recessive alleles are involved. Where both gene-gene interactions and non-genetic factors in prenatal and postnatal life contribute to the disease phenotype, the expression of a single causative gene is improbable (Bittles & Black, 2010).

Numerous different directions have been followed in research and into the ***treatment of stuttering***, with varying attitudinal differences across cultures. The nature of treatment depends upon the age, severity and attitude of the PWS. Speech therapist have developed established treatments that focuses on breathing pattern, slow/prolongated speech, relaxation techniques and reading complex sentences loudly. Behavioral, cognitive, pharmacological and related treatments are available for stuttering (Bothe *et al.*, 2006) and, besides speech-language pathologists, in India psychologists, psychiatrists and practitioners of alternative systems of medicine also treat the disorder (Subramanian & Prabhu, 2005).

2.6 CAUSES OF STUTTERING

Stuttering is caused due to miscommunication between their premotor and mechanical process. The miscommunication happens only at the moment of speech indicating that they do not have any problem with premotor process (as they know what they want to say). A variety of factors influence stuttering but the etiology still remains obscure. Various research studies were published in neurological and genetic perspectives to decode the etiology of stuttering.

2.6.1 NEUROLOGICAL PERSPECTIVES IN STUTTERING

The underlying cause for stuttering had been contemplated since antiquity (Orton, 1927) on abnormal functional lateralization of cortical connections (Chang, 2014). Despite early speculation only in mid 1980s, studies focused on brain structure and function of individuals with stuttering. The advanced brain imaging techniques that visualized the activity of the intact brain yielded significant results. Even with the use of most advanced neuroimaging techniques we are not able to find any objective markers specific for individuals with stuttering. This is due to the fact that the brains of individuals with stuttering do not exhibit any gross abnormality.

Most studies have examined adults who might have developed various motoric or emotional reactions associated with stuttering. Very few studies have examined children close to onset. However it is important to remember that our understanding on brain development have increased and the fact that brain plasticity can be influenced for speech fluency (Chang, 2014).

Overactive right hemisphere was observed in adults who stutter (Fox *et al.*, 1996) but no such laterality differences was observed in children indicating right hemisphere activity may have developed possibly as a reaction to stuttering and not the basis for stuttering (Chang *et al.*, 2011). Since the children were 6-12 years of age there is still chance of capturing reactions to stuttering. Observing children close to onset will resolve such issues (Choo *et al.*, 2012).

Wu *et al.*, (1997) also investigated the role of the dopamine system in stuttering. They found significant increases in dopamine uptake activity in the cortical and subcortical regions that are associated with speech. Stuttering subjects showed considerably **higher uptake** than normal controls in **medial prefrontal, deep orbital, insular and auditory cortex, extended amygdala and caudate tail**. This finding is also consistent with earlier findings of decreased metabolic activity in many of the same regions in stutterers (Wu *et al.,* 1995; Braun *et al.,* 1997) due to excess dopamine having an inhibitory effect on regional cerebral glucose metabolism.

In a study by (Lan *et al.*, 2009) the association between dopaminergic genes (*DRD2* and *SLC6A3*) and stuttering among Han Chinese (112) was evaluated by determining the allele frequency of 5 SNPs (rs2617604, rs28364997, rs28364998 in *SLC6A3* and rs6275, rs6277 in *DRD2*). Presence of C allele at rs6277 SNP in *DRD2* was associated with increased susceptibility to stuttering. However two other studies (Drayna & Kang, 2011; Montag *et al.*, 2012) did not find any association of rs6277 in *DRD2* with stuttering. But Montag and his colleagues outlined the importance of endophenotype (personality dimension neuroticism) and showed that rs6277 influences stuttering by its influence on neuroticism. Thus, the role of dopamine as a causative for stuttering has been reported variably and remains inconclusive.

In a study by Chang et.al., (2013) the interaction of brain regions when children at rest was studied using fMRI. They observed **decreased functional connectivity in two neural circuits: inferior frontal -motor-auditory circuit** and **SMA-putamen**. It suggests that CWS have deficiency in motor planning, execution and timing of self-initiated production of speech. The study also observed sex differences that showed decreased connectivity in both boys and girls in SMA-putamen and only boys in IFG-motor-STG circuits. It is possible that **auditory-motor circuit could support recovery** (as more females recover) but requires confirmation from longitudinal studies (Chang & Zhu, 2013). These results provide evidence for significant differences in brain connectivity at very early age in children. In sum the neural networks that support normal timing of self-initiated motor sequences is affected in CWS.

2.6.2 GENETIC PERSPECTIVES OF STUTTERING

The underlying causes were studied intensively in the past four decades that steadily accumulated the involvement of genetic factors. **Familial aggregation** or clustering among the families of individuals with stuttering was observed since 1939 by Nelson and many others later. Consistently all reported higher proportion (4-6 times) of affected relatives in families of individuals with stuttering than in control families (Yairi, Ambrose & Cox, 1996). Such familial aggregation could be due to genes or environment or both.

The classical approaches that established the genetic nature of the disorder are **twin and adoption studies**. In the past 40 years nine twin studies were published all of which concluded higher concordance in monozygotic than dizygotic twins indicating a strong evidence for genetic nature of the disorder. However the concordance was <1 and heritability estimates were varied (42-85%) indicating that genetic factors alone does not contribute to stuttering (Godai & Tatarelli, 1976; Howie, 1981; Andrews *et al.*, 1991; Felsenfeld *et al.*, 2000; Ooki, 2005;Dworzynski *et al.*, 2007; van Beijsterveldt, Felsenfeld & Boomsma, 2010; Fagnani *et al.*, 2011; Rautakoski *et al.*, 2012). Adoption studies were very few with statistical limitations but still tend to disprove that stuttering develops by listening to their parents with stuttering (Bloodstein, 1961; Felsenfeld & Plomin, 1997).

There were several epidemiological studies in stuttering that sought to explain the mode of inheritance. **Segregation analysis** was applied to pedigrees with positive family history to understand the pattern of inheritance of a trait within families. In stuttering families several models (**multifactorial polygenic** - many genes with small effect and also environmental components, **single locus model** - one gene with large effect and number of genes with small effect and environmental component, **autosomal dominant locus** etc. were proposed and the mode of inheritance was unlikely to be in Mendelian fashion as observed by several studies (Kidd *et al.,* 1981; MacFarlane *et al.*, 1991; Ambrose *et al*, 1993; Viswanath *et al.,* 2000; Viswanath *et al.,* 2004; Riaz *et al.*, 2005; Wittke-Thompson *et al.*, 2007). All the above studies provided conflicting evidence on the mode of inheritance. However, with the strong evidence of heritability to stuttering justified an advance from statistical to biological genetics.

Linkage studies in stuttering

Mapping genes is the greatest challenge in stuttering as it is a complex disorder where genetic dissection is made difficult due to gene-gene, gene-environment interactions, genetic heterogeneity, gender bias, incomplete penetrance and phenocopies. In order to identify the causative genes, several linkage studies were performed in numerous multiplex families.

A first genome-wide linkage survey was on a genetically isolated Hutterite population with stuttering supported linkage on chromosomes 1, 13 and 16 (Cox & Yairi,

2000). Following this (Shugart *et al.*, 2004) performed a linkage study using nonparametric method on 68 general outbred families from North American and Europe. Evidence of linkage was observed on chromosome 18 that harbors interesting candidate genes in desmoglein/desmocolin family and neuronal cadherin 2 gene that helps in cell-cell communication and cell adhesion. Such communications are found to be important in the neurons involved in the production of speech.

Riaz *et al.*, (2005) employed 46 highly inbred multiplex families from Pakistan consisting of 144 affected and 55 unaffected. They also used non parametric method and found consistent evidence of linkage on chromosome 12 with a LOD score as high as 4.61 suggesting that this locus may contain a gene with large effect resulting in stuttering, in this population.

Very close to this report in the following year (Suresh *et al.*, 2006), performed linkage on 100 European families with 252 persistent and 45 recovered individuals with stuttering and reported suggestive linkage on chromosome 9, analyzing both persistent and recovered stuttering individuals; but on chromosome 15 when considering only persistent stuttering individuals. They also identified a sex specific signal on chromosome 7 on analyzing males and chromosome 12 on females, suggesting significant sex effects.

Another interesting linkage study by (Wittke-Thompson *et al.*, 2007) on Hutterite founder population with traceable 232-person genealogy, showed linkage on chromosomes 3, 13 and 15 for stuttering. Meta-analysis combining their data with European families showed a nominal linkage on chromosomes 2 and 5. Even though these linkage signals could not meet the genome-wide criterion for significance some stronger signals overlie the linkage mapping signals reported previously for speech and language disorders. In all the above five studies, only Riaz *et al.*, (2005) was able to get significant linkage score as they focused on consanguineous families owing to increased homozygosity, bringing the rare alleles together.

Identification of the first gene GNPTAB for stuttering on chromosome 12

The 10kb linkage region identified by Riaz *et al.*, (2005) on chromosome 12 set the stage for Kang *et al.*, (2010) to conduct a fine mapping, that revealed 87 genes in the region of which 45 were taken up for sequencing. The mutation that co-segregated in the family was Glu1200Lys a highly conserved mutation which substituted lysine in place of glutamic acid in *GNPTAB* gene (OMIM#607840). This was the first gene that was implicated in stuttering.

Nevertheless, the segregation of *GNPTAB* mutation was not perfect in the family, as three affected individuals lacked the mutation while one unaffected had the mutation. The former situation was explained by the phenomenon of genetic heterogeneity and nongenetic causes of stuttering that might have resulted in such phenocopies. The later situation was attributed to naturally recovering phenomenon especially in women.

Three other independent Pakistani families also carried the same *GNPTAB* gene mutation when sequenced. Screening *GNPTAB* gene in unrelated stuttering cases revealed that 5/123 Pakistani and 1/270 North American-Britain cases carried same mutation. This mutation was absent in 276 Causcasian controls but was present in one normal Pakistan individual in heterozygous condition (Kang et al., 2010a). Subsequently (*GNPTAB)* p.Glu1200Lys mutation was shown to be the founder mutation having a unique haplotype and the age of mutation was estimated to be 14,300 years (Fedyna *et al.*, 2011). Further investigations led to the identification of three other *GNPTAB* gene mutations that were not observed in controls (Kang *et al.*, 2010). They concluded that mutations in *GNPTAB* can cause stuttering. *GNPTAB* gene encodes GlcNAc-1-phosphotransferase alpha and beta subunits that is known to be involved in lysosomal targeting pathway.

Identification of two more putative genes *GNPTG* and *NAGPA* on chromosome 16 in the same lysosomal targeting pathway

GNPTG (encoding the gamma subunit of GlcNAc-1-phosphotransferase enzyme) and *NAGPA* (N-acetylglucosamine-1-phosphodiester alpha-Nacetylglucosaminidase), are two other functionally related genes that also provided additional evidence for their role in stuttering in the same pathway. Three different mutations in *GNPTG* gene in 4 stuttering individuals and 3 different mutations in *NAGPA* gene in 6 unrelated cases were identified but not in any of the controls. All the mutations identified are present in the highly conserved regions.

Thus, the three genes *GNPTAB*, *GNPTG* and *NAGPA* became the biological candidate genes for stuttering. A strong connection was established between stuttering and four mutations in *GNPTAB*, three in *GNPTG* and three in *NAGPA* gene. Table 1 summarizes the distribution of these mutations in Pakistani and North American-Britain cases elucidated in Kang *et al.*, (2010) study.

Though this finding of these genes also provides a possible neurochemical basis for white matter abnormalities observed in stuttering (lysosomes participates in protein trafficking that is crucial for biogenesis and also maintenance of myelin sheaths) the effect of the mutations in neural cell biology is still unexplored (Büchel & Watkins, 2010).

Table 1: Distribution of different mutations in *GNPTAB*, *GNPTG* & *NAGPA* genes implicated in stuttering

GENE/EXON	MUTATION	AMINO ACID CHANGE
GNPTAB		
Exon9	c.961A > G	p.Ser321Gly
Exon11	c.1363 G > T	p.Ala455Ser
Exon13	c.1875 C > G	p.Phe624Leu
Exon19	c.3598 G > A	p.Glu1200Lys
GNPTG		
Exon1	c.11_19dup	p.Leu 5_Arg7dup
Exon2	c.74 C > A	p.Ala25Glu
Exon9	c.688 C > G	p.Leu230Val
NAGPA		
Exon2	c.252 C > G	p.His84Gln
Exon6	c.982 C > T	p.Arg328Cys
Exon10	c.1538_1553del	p.Phe513SerfsX113

Source: Adapted from Kang et.al., 2010

Enzymology of the lysosomal targeting Mannose-6- phosphate (M6P) pathway

Lysosomal hydrolases are synthesized in the RER (Rough endoplasmic reticulum) and transported through Golgi to lysosome by transport vesicles. The lysosomal enzymes are recognized by a unique marker M6P that are added to N-linked oligosaccharides of the enzymes as they pass from *cis* to *trans* Golgi.

The M6P marker is generated by two enzymes:

i. GlcNAc-1-phosphotransferase is a hexameric complex encoded by two genes, *GNPTAB* (membrane bound α/β-precursor) & GNPTG (soluble γ subunit) (Tiede et al., 2005). The enzyme produced is assembled in the ER and is transported to Golgi in inactive form where it is proteolytically cleaved to active α and β subunits. γ subunit binds to α subunit and enhances the enzyme activity (Figure 5).

ii. α-N-acetylglucosamine-1-phosphodiesterα-N-acetylglucosaminidase encoded by *NAGPA*

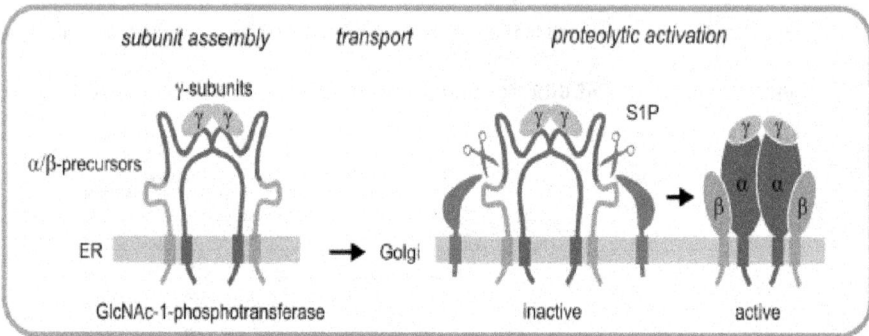

Figure 5: **Membrane bound GlcNAc-1-phosphotransferase complex activation** (Source: Velho et al., 2019)

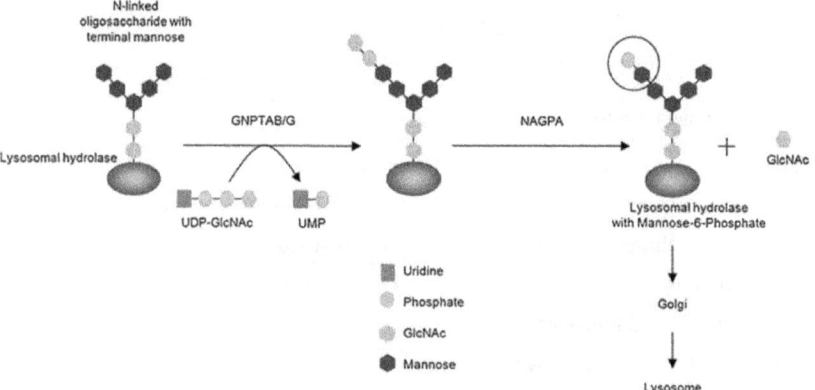

Figure 6: M6P tagging for transport of lysosomal enzyme (Source: Kang & Drayna, 2011)

The Figure 6 depicts the two-step process of addition of the marker.
a) In the first step phosphotransferase transfers GlcNAc-1-phosphate residue from UDP GlcNAc to C6 position of terminal mannose residue of hydrolases.
b) Removal of terminal GlcNAc by Phosphodiesterase also called UCE (uncovering enzyme) that exposes the M6P recognition signal.

These enzymes are recognized by cation dependent or independent transmembrane M6P receptors that bind to M6P marked hydrolases on the luminal side of golgi membrane and to adaptins in cytosolic side. Thus, the receptors help to pack the hydrolases in clathrin coated vesicles and transfer them form trans Golgi to endosomes that becomes mature lysosomes. The hydrolases that are delivered digest the endocyted material.

Additional linkage loci identified on chromosomes 3q, 16q and 10q

Parametric linkage analysis in two newly ascertained consanguineous Pakistani families identified two more new linkage loci on chromosome 3q13.2–3q13.33 with maximum two point LOD score of 4.23 (Raza, Riazuddin, & Drayna, 2010) and 16q12.1–16q23.1 with a multipoint LOD score of 4.42 (Raza *et al.*, 2012) under recessive model.

Genome wide linkage scan on 43 Brazilian multiplex families with persistent stuttering was performed by Domingues *et al.*, (2014). A significant linkage with a combined maximum single-point LOD score of 4.02 and a multipoint LOD score of 4.28 on chromosome 10q21 for two families under dominant model was reported.

Identification of *CNTNAP2* as another candidate gene in a syndromic stuttering case

Petrin et.al., (2010) reported on a Brazilian case with an intricate set of speech and language difficulties in addition to stuttering. A 10 Mb micro deletion on chromosome 7q33-35 disrupts the first three exons of *CNTNAP2* gene including a deletion of binding site for the transcription factor *FOXP2*. *CNTNAP2* gene was previously implicated in language disorders (Poot *et al.*, 2009) and ASD with speech delay (Poot *et al.*, 2010) and belongs to the same pathway as *FOXP2* which is also extensively studied in the context of verbal dyspraxia. All the above genetic studies are compiled in the Table 2.

Table 2: Compilation of genetic studies in numerous multiplex families worldwide (2002-2017)

Genetic studies	Population	Chromosomal region	Statistical strength and gene identification
Cox N, Yairi E., 2002	Hutterites North Dakota	1	suggestive
		13	suggestive
Shugart et. al., 2004	North America and Europe	18p	suggestive
		18q	suggestive
Riaz et. al., 2005	Pakistani families	**12q**	**Highly significant**
Suresh et.al., 2006	Americans (European descent), Swedish and Israelis	**2q**	significant
		7q	suggestive
		9p	suggestive
		12q	suggestive
		13q	suggestive
		15q	suggestive
		20p	suggestive
		21q	**Highly significant**
Wittke-Thompson et,al., 2007	Hutterites South Dakota	3q	suggestive
		13q	suggestive
		15q	suggestive
		9q	suggestive
		3q	suggestive
		13q	suggestive
		2q	suggestive
		5q	suggestive
Lan et. al., 2009	Han Chinese	*DRD2* and *SLC6A3*	Association of DRD2
Kang et. al., 2010	Pakistan	Fine mapping of 12q	*GNPTAB*
Raza et. al., 2010	Pakistan	3q (*DRD3*)	**Highly significant** No variation
Petrin et.al., 2010	Brazil	7q	*CNTNAP2*
Kang et,al., 2011	Brazil	*DRD2*	*No association*
Raza et. al., 2012	Pakistan	16q	**Highly significant**
Raza et. al., 2013	Camaroon, Africa	2p	**Highly significant**
		3p	significant
		3q	**Highly significant**
		14q	**Highly significant**
		15q	**Highly significant**
Domingues et. al., 2014	Brazil	10q	significant
Raza et. al., 2015	Camaroon, Africa	Fine mapping of 15q	*AP4E1*

Genetic studies	Population	Chromosomal region	Statistical strength and gene identification
Kazemi et.al., 2017	Iran	Replication study	*GNPTAB, GNPTG, NAGPA*

Adapted and modified from Domingues and Drayna, 2017

Genome-wide association study of persistent developmental stuttering

Only one genome-wide association study (GWAS) on 122 stuttering individuals of European descent is available (Kraft, 2010). Although no significant GWAS hits were found, nine suggestive candidate genes (*FADS2, PLXNA4, CTNNA3, ARNT2, EYA2, PCSK5, SLC24A3, FMN1, ADARB2*) involved in neural pathways were identified in persistent developmental stuttering, together with a SNP (rs2573111) upstream of a small non-coding RNA (RNU6-259P). These genes are involved in neural development, function and behaviour (Kraft & Yairi, 2011).

Whole exome sequencing study in a family with stuttering

. An earlier linkage study (Raza *et al.*, 2013) on a large polygamous kindred of 71 members from Camaroon in which 33 were affected identified multiple chromosomal regions on 2, 3, 14 and 15 in different branches of the family. Initial linkage scan could not identify any linkage but only after dividing the pedigree into five sub pedigrees, linkage evidence was observed on 3q and 15q previously reported loci. Additionally, 2p,3p and 14q novel loci and two different regions on 15q were also observed. This study indicated that multiple genes may be involved in causing the phenotype. In this backdrop with the advent of high throughput NGS technologies the family initially linked to chromosome 15 were revisited for fine mapping.

Whole exome sequencing identified two rare coding variants (p. Val517Ile in exon 14 and p. Glu801Lys in exon 18) in Adaptor Protein complex 4 Epsilon subunit 1 (*AP4E1*) gene that co-segregated with persistent developmental stuttering. It is involved in protein sorting at the trans-Golgi network. The study was further extended to 96 unrelated stuttering individuals from Cameroon that identified the same two rare mutations in 2 affected individuals but not in 94 Cameroon controls nor in the public database.

In the third leg of extension more unrelated Cameroon (93), Pakistan (132) and North America (711) stuttering individuals were sequenced for *AP4E1* gene. Twenty-three additional rare variants were observed resulting in a **combined frequency of 3.7%** (35/936) at significantly higher rate, than in population matched controls (9/558) (Cameroon 94; Pakistan 96; North America 368). Variations observed includes missense, deletions, duplications, insertions, frameshift stop codons. All mutation were in heterozygous condition in the affected (Raza *et al*., 2015). The m4 subunit of AP4 interacts with NAGPA establishing a possible link with lysosomal targeting pathway that is previously implicated with stuttering.

To summarize in the so far reported studies, either significant or suggestive evidence for linkage is distributed throughout the chromosomal complement (2/3rd) except for chromosomes 4, 6, 8, 11,17, 19, 22, X and Y (Figure A1). Only two studies (Kang *et al*., 2010; Raza *et al*., 2015) marked in the figure led to the identification of genes. Compilation of genes potentially involved in speech and language disorders are listed in Table A1 (Guerra & Cacabelos, 2019; Szalontai & Csiszár, 2013).

2.7 ELUCIDATION OF THE PATHOLOGY OF IMPLICATED GENES IN STUTTERING

With the identification of genes, the primary goal of stuttering was to identify the neuropathology underlying the disorder. Stuttering individuals carrying mutations in the four currently identified genes, reviewed above do not display any neurological deficits other than stuttering. Hence it was hypothesized that pathogenicity of mutations is restricted to speech specific neurons. Identifying those neurons require a tractable animal model that led to the construction of mouse models. Mice display Ultrasonic vocalizations that are well characterized and under genetic control. In a study (Barnes *et al*., 2016), mice was engineered to carry p.Glu1176Lys mutation which is the mouse homolog of human Glu1200Lys mutation in *GNPTAB* gene. The mice did not have any obvious abnormalities and they grow, breed, produce litters normally and had normal behaviour. Their vocalizations were similar to normal littermates (8-day old pup) but there was significant difference in timing of vocalization (longer pauses) similar to human stuttering phenotype.

Two other GNPTAB gene mutations Ser321Gly and Ala455Ser were engineered in mice that displayed vocalization deficits (8-day old pup) similar to human stuttering. Immunohistochemistry of Ser321Gly homozygous mice showed a decreased staining in astrocytes compared to wild-type, while cerebellar Purkinje cells, microglial cells, oligodendrocytes and dopaminergic neurons did not show any significant difference in staining. DTI showed deficits in corpus callosum. Cell-specific Cre-drivers in Ser321Gly knockout mice showed that only astrocytes displayed vocalization deficits. These findings indicate that abnormality lies in astrocytes of corpus callosum thereby supporting the hypothesis of deficits in interhemispheric communication (Han *et al.*, 2019).

The genes identified were functionally related but the mutations reported in stuttering does not completely abolish the function of the enzyme but only reduces its activity. Hence how a single mutation in common housekeeping gene can result in stuttering is still a mystery. One possibility hypothesized was that neuron specific for speech, are sensitive to accumulation of waste due to missing lysosomal enzymes causing the morbidity. But they were not able to delineate speech specific neurons nor did they observe any evidence of accumulation of waste. Another possibility may be those genes have yet another function that is unidentified (www.sciencemag.com).

2.8 STUTTERING GENES WERE PREVIOUSLY IMPLICATED IN A RARE LYSOSOMAL STORAGE DISORDER - MUCOLIPIDOSIS

Mucolipidosis (ML) is a set of inherited metabolic disorders that affect the normal turnover of various waste materials within cells. It is characterized by disorders of skeletal system, joints, motor system, heart, spleen and liver. Mucolipidosis is classified from I to IV. ML II is the fatal form whose symptoms are evident from birth caused by *GNPTAB* gene. ML III occurs at a later age with longer life caused by both *GNPTAB* and *GNPTG* genes hence named as ML III α/β and ML III γ (is a milder form) respectively (Cathey *et al.*, 2008).

Defective GlcNAc1phosphotransferase found in the cells of ML II/III affected persons mis sorts the lysosomal enzymes resulting in hypersecretion of it in the extracellular environment. Due to deficiency of lysosomal enzymes in lysosomes there is accumulation of undigested macromolecules in lysosome that impairs homeostasis as well as cellular function (Kollmann *et al.*, 2010).

It was elegantly recognized by Kang et.al., (2010) that the mutations in *GNPTAB* gene identified in stuttering were the ones that were already established in mucolipidosis. Yet the stuttering individuals did not display any typical symptoms of mucolipidosis. The pathogenic role of these genes in stuttering was supported by the fact that they are (i) identified only in stuttering individuals (ii) the mutations were conserved and (iii) occurred in a well-defined metabolic pathway. (Kang *et al.*, 2010). The location of type of mutations were also compared with the mutations identified in mucolpidosis. So far 81 different variants were identified in the stuttering individuals of which 75 (92.6%) were missense mutations. The difference in the mutations observed in stuttering and mucolipidosis is summarized below (Table 3).

Table 3: Overview of mutations in stuttering vs. mucolipidosis

STUTTERING	MUCOLIPIDOSIS
Typically, heterozygous	Homozygous
Typical missense	Many null alleles
Reduction of enzymatic function	No enzymatic function
Mutations in mucolipidosis are at different sites than stuttering	Mutations in stuttering are at different sites than mucolipidosis

Adapted from Frigerio-Domingues & Drayna, 2017

Compilation of variants so far reported in mucolipidosis is given in figures A3 and A3. It was suggested that mutations in *GNPTAB* and *GNPTG* genes that cause stuttering is different from those that lead to MLII/III. This hypothesis was supported by the fact that of the variants identified in *GNPTAB* and *GNPTG* genes in stuttering individuals only four was previously reported in mucolipidosis (Figure 7).

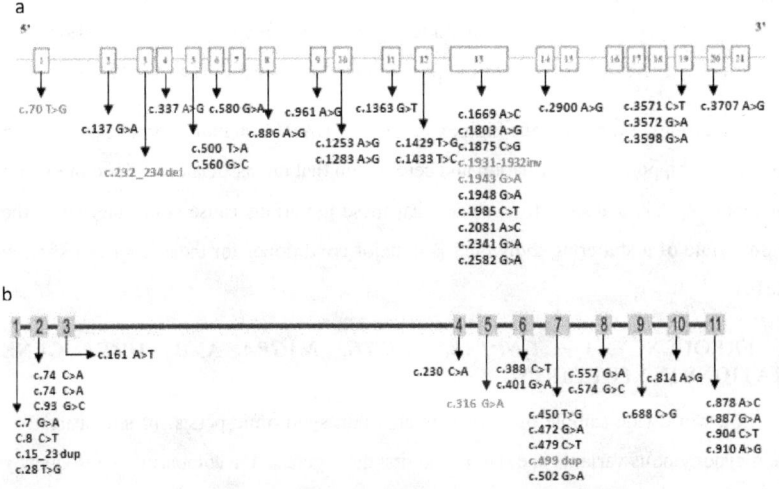

Figure 7: (a) *GNPTAB* (b) *GNPTG* gene exonic mutation spectrum so far reported in stuttering. Red colour variants indicates the ones also reported in mucolipidosis

NAGPA was so far not implicated in any disorders including mucolipidosis though it is acting in the same pathway of *GNPTAB* and *GNPTG* genes. This was explained by Chavez and his collaborators (Chavez *et al.*, 2007) and also confirmed by Boonen *et al.*, (2009) in vivo study, that UCE deficiencies probably may not be lethal because cation independent M6P receptor was able to bind with GlcNAC-P-Man diesters but with low affinity than M6P monoesters. Hence even in the absence of UCE the hydrolases could be transported to the lysosomes that is sufficient in preventing phenotypes of lysosomal storage disorder (Coutinho, Prata & Alves, 2012).

The effect of mutations identified in stuttering on phosphotransferase and UCE were not examined so far, and so it is possible that the mutations may or may not be detrimental. Since the role of *GNPTAB* and *GNPTG* genes are controversial and also well studied in mucolipidosis, only *NAGPA* mutations (p. Arg328Cys and p. F513SfsX113) were evaluated biochemically. It was found that mutation in *NAGPA* disrupt proper folding with rapid degradation in ER that reduces the enzyme activity by 50% (Lee *et al.*, 2011). It is not clearly understood how reduced activities leads to stuttering mutations. However it is understood that mutations identified in stuttering has less effects on protein function than mutations in MLII/III that leads to loss of protein function (Kang & Drayna, 2012).

Interestingly on finding the high expression of *GNPTG* in mouse brain especially in hippocampus, hippocampal formation and cerebellum that are associated with emotion and motor function, it is plausible to consider that these mutations cause stuttering, since the emotional state of a stuttering individual is a major conditioner for their severity (Kang *et al.*, 2010).

2.9 FREQUENCY OF *GNPTAB*, *GNPTG*, *NAGPA* AND *AP4E1* GENE MUTATIONS IN STUTTERING

In a worldwide sample of 1013 unrelated non syndromic persistent stuttering, 164 had non-synonymous variants in either of the first three genes. On comparing the frequency of these variants with the public databases, stuttering individuals had higher rate than controls (Raza *et al.*, 2016). The contribution of mutations in *GNPTAB* gene was 8.6% (87/1013), *GNPTG* was 4.4% (45/1013) and NAGPA 3.2% (32/1013) resulting in a combined frequency of 16%. (Raza *et al.*, 2016). The combined contribution of mutations in the four genes *GNPTAB, GNPTG, NAGPA* and *AP4E1* to stuttering was thus estimated to be 20% (Domingues & Drayna, 2017).

A study by Kazemi et.al., (2018) used homozygosity mapping and Sanger sequencing to investigate the reported variations in the three genes *(GNPTAB, GNPTG* and *NAGPA)* among 25 Iranian families. They observed 14 variations in these three genes, of which 3 variations cosegregated in the stuttering families. It includes a novel intronic variant (g.10985G>A) in *GNPTG* gene and 2 bp deletion (c.3503_3504delTC) and a missense mutation (c.2094A>G) in *GNPTAB* gene. The importance of the implicated genes for stuttering is reflected on its replication in this study, further confirming its role in stuttering.

A recent study by Benito-Aragón *et al.,* (2020) had elucidated that *GNPTG* – a gene involved in the mannose-6-phosphate lysosomal targeting pathways – was significantly co-localized with the stuttering cortical network based on functional connectivity MRI and graph theory. This study had utilized a spatial similarity analysis approach that elucidated the topology of the stuttering cortical network by intersecting with genetic expression levels of previously reported genes for stuttering from the protein-coding transcriptome data of the Allen Human Brain Atlas.

2.10 ROLE OF *FOXP2* GENE IN STUTTERING

A unique entry into neuromuscular mechanisms influencing the acquisition speech and language was unlocked by *FOXP2* which is the first gene identified in severe form of speech and language disorder (SPCH1[MIM 602081]) (Fisher *et al.*, 2001). It is located in 7q31 and encodes a transcription factor involved early in embryogenesis during the development of neural structures that are important in speech and language. The *FOXP2* gene regulates the embryonic development of striatum that comprises of basal ganglia and its associated subcortical structures. Mutations in *FOXP2* gene is implicated in verbal dyspraxia that is characterized by orofacial motor, comprehension, cognitive and speech production deficits in most of the members of KE family (Fisher *et al.*, 1998; MacDermot *et al.*, 2005). Neural expression of *FOXP2* early in brain development in both mice and human was determined by (Lai et.al., 2003). *FOXP2* deficiency disrupts basal ganglia and subcortical structure development leading to deficits in speech production (Lieberman, 2006).

A possible relation between stuttering and basal ganglia was proposed (Caruso, 1991; Molt, 1999; Alm, 2004). Instances when there is an absence of stuttering gives an important clue of the underlying motor dysfunction. When a PWS follows a beat or singing there is an absence of stuttering which is known as the 'rhythm effect'. This effect is explained as an instance where the external timing cues, masks the characteristic dysfunction of basal ganglia motor circuits but the problem persists in performing motor sequences on their own. Basal ganglia provides go signals for segments of motor sequences like syllables in speech (Alm, 2004). The role of basal ganglia in stuttering is further iterated by (i) lesions in basal ganglia in acquired stuttering (Ludlow et.al., 1987), (ii) dopamine regulating the basal ganglia and (iii) by the fact that basal ganglia motor disorders worsen in stress and improve in relaxed conditions.

But motor circuits involved in striatum is critical in general for movement sequence and not specifically for speech, however both KE and stuttering individuals do not exhibit severe impairment in movements other than speech. Also, interesting differences in speech disruptions in KE and PWS were observed. PWS have difficulty in initiation of a word and on specific words but often experience periods of fluency. Speech difficulties in KE family is more persistent and does not improve with practice (Watkins, 2011). Inspite of similarities there is still no evidence for the role of *FOXP2* with stuttering.

Cerebellum is majorly composed of Purkinje cells that plays major role in control of motor function. Deficits in these brain regions were prominent in the cells that carry *FOXP2* mutations (Fujita et.al., 2008). However in a mice that carried Ser321Gly homozygous stuttering mutation the Purkinje cells had normal staining that signifies the view that *FOXP2* does not have role in stuttering and is both pathologically and genetically distinct from verbal dyspraxia (Han *et al.*, 2019).

2.11 TREATMENT IN STUTTERING

Genetic research in stuttering has identified few genes but is not found in majority of PWS and is best described as a polygenic disorder. The discovery of these genes are interesting as it implicates a molecular suspect that is already implicated in the lysosomal storage disorder. Since the genes control broad functions for metabolic function producing a knockout would be fatal and hence gene therapies is far from reach.

Both anatomic and functional studies implicate differences in grey and white matter, connectivity between speech language and motor regions and functional differences in speech-language processing. These differences are found to be casual rather than adaption that were confirmed from studies in children. These findings shed light on differences in response of treatment among PWS. One such evidence is typical cortical asymmetry observed in normal individuals that was absent in some PWS. This particular group benefitted well to **Altered Auditory Feedback (AAF).**

The severity of stuttered speech often does not indicate the depth of struggle the individual with stuttering faces owing to the impact of the disorder. It not only has **behavioural and cognitive impact** but also has adverse effect on the quality of life. It also has interfered with the relationships with the family, particularly parents, siblings and their life partners. Hence therapy not only involves the actual strategy for fluent speech but also requires **psychological support** that reduces their anxiety and negative pressures (Beilby, 2014). The treatment focuses on relaxation techniques, slow speech, read the sentences loudly and in case of any block relaxing with deep breath or use alternate words.

Biology is not the destiny. Learning and **automatizing** new speaking patterns can **'rewire'** the brain circuits for speech production. Thus, treatment of stuttering concentrates not only on core and associated motor behaviours but also on cognitive reactions. There were arguments to which aspect should be targeted first. It is also difficult to treat core behaviours without working on aspects of affective and cognitive features. Also, it is difficult to determine the outcome of therapy as there are no objective measures for cognitive features as there is for measuring the core behaviours (SSI). Overall Assessment of the Speaker's Experience of Stuttering (**OASES**) by (Yaruss & Quesal, 2006) for wide age range and **KiddyCAT** (Commercially available test) for preschoolers are now available to measures different aspects like functional impact on life style, cognitive/emotional measures and communication attitudes (Vanryckeghem, Brutten & Hernandez, 2005). Peer reactions (**bullying and teasing**) are also accounted (Blood & Blood, 2016). Further it was hard to document the variability in fluency in different social situations in real life than clinical settings. For this a novel approach called **virtual reality** was investigated by Shelley Brundage and colleagues for evaluating fluency in various real-life settings (Brundage *et al.*, 2006). There are also **self-help groups** for stuttering where they interact and share each other their experiences and managing strategy in speaking situations (https://stammer.in/- The Indian stammering association-TISA).

A highly published and thoroughly evaluated therapy for stuttering in young children was **Lidcombe Program** that was evaluated and implemented in Australia. For older children two approaches **fluency shaping** and **stuttering modification** that are often integrated, were recognized (Ratner, 2010).

Pharmacological interventions were adopted for stuttering to improve motor coordination and anxiety. Hence medications prescribed in managing psychiatric illness were used to treat stuttering. Some of them are haloperidol, risperidone, olanzapine, clomipramine, alprazolam etc., but in general, these drug treatments were not considered effective or sufficiently safe (Friedlander *et al.*, 2004).

Since stuttering is intertwined with physiological, emotional and anxiety factors and negative experiences in speaking occasions aggravate stuttering, **yoga interventions** were also suggested. Yoga encompass asanas (poses), pranayama (breathing exercise), and meditation (Sherman, 2012) that induces PNS activation (limbic regions) and suppress SNS. PNS is responsible for relaxed state, decrease heart rate and blood pressure whereas SNS is opposite for stress response (Pramanik *et al.*, 2009). Yoga intervention can be sound complementary approach for reducing the anxiety and stress that accompanies stuttering in conjunction traditional therapies. However only few studies are available (Kauffman, 2016).

The **effect of Fluency shaping therapies include:** reduction in right hemispheric over activation, normalization of basal ganglia activity, reactivation of left hemispheric cortex (Neumann *et al.*, 2005; Giraud *et al.*, 2008). However, a stabilized therapeutic outcome requires repeated training and refresher sessions. Relateralization of speech network is therefore only transient and overall insufficient repair process. The current absence of a definitive etiology has slowed advancements in the clinical sphere of the disorder.

2.12 CURRENT CHALLENGES

All the genes that were identified so far point to a single intracellular trafficking process that are promising concepts in neurological disorders. Initially such deficits were recognized as rare Mendelian disorders but now are found to be important in complex disorders as well. Till date only two linkage studies led to the identification of the genes and other significant linkage loci reported on chromosomes 2, 3p,3q, 10, 14 and 16 still remained unanswered. Identifying these genes are challenging. Since linkage and association studies are time-consuming and progress gradually, whole exome sequencing is now taking the center stage that would soon improve the process of identifying more genes that are associated with stuttering mechanism.

AIM

The overall aim is to study **the genetic epidemiology and determine the molecular basis of developmental stuttering**

SPECIFIC OBJECTIVES

1. To determine the prevalence of childhood stuttering in Tamil Nadu
2. To characterize developmental stuttering by observable behaviors and identify the risk factors associated with stuttering
3. To assess the genetic component in stuttering
4. To investigate the genetic predisposition of stuttering due to *DRD2 Taq*IA polymorphism
5. To completely sequence ten specific exons from three previously reported/implicated genes for stuttering *viz.*, *GNPTAB*, *GNPTG* and *NAGPA*.
6. To comprehensively screen selected multiplex families, using exome sequencing to determine the role of known and other new genes involved in stuttering.

CHAPTER 3

METHODOLOGY

PHASE I - GENETIC EPIDEMIOLOGY

Ethical clearance for this study was approved by the Institutional Human Ethical Committee of University of Madras (Approval No: PGIBMS/CO/Tara/Human Ethical/2005-06/850 dated 15.7.2005) (Appendix- 1).

3.1 DATA FROM SCHOOLS FOR THE ASSESSMENT OF PREVALENCE

Totally 100 schools were approached during a period of five years, of which 97 schools consented to participate in the screening for stuttering. Overall, 74,544 students were screened and 342 children with stuttering (CWS) were identified. The schools were recruited from two cities, Chennai (n=78) and Salem (n=19) (Figure 8) that hail from both government and private educational sectors and from various socio-economic strata.

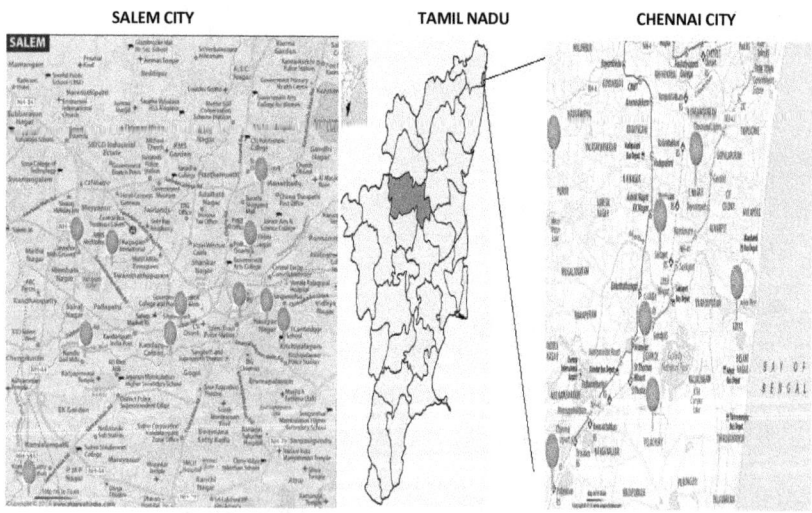

Figure 8: Salem and Chennai city maps showing the location of the schools screened

3.1.1 Proband ascertainment and assessment

The principals of the schools were approached with an official letter (Appendix 2) describing the proposed study and its objectives. Similarly, the *class teacher* was also elaborately oriented about the study. In India, though many teachers teach various subjects, there will be a designated class teacher who co-ordinates, prepares the progress reports and interacts extensively with every student of that class and their parents. In other words, the class teacher has maximum interaction with each student in multiple dimensions and meets them almost every day. This was the rationale in approaching class teachers to get the preliminary reference.

Based on their personal assessment, the class teachers were asked to provide a list of students with any slightest perceived problem in communication and speaking, including those who were constantly reluctant to speak. The investigators were trained by the speech therapist to identify CWS during the initial screening.

3.1.2 Characterization of speech

Those children with suspected problems in speech, who were shortlisted in the first phase in accordance with the teachers' referral, were further intensively analyzed for speech and non-speech behaviors that are associated with stuttering, in a dedicated room allocated by the school authorities. These students were systematically evaluated through face-to-face interview. Three tasks were given to each of the students: casual conversation to elicit spontaneous speech, followed by a reading (Appendix-3) and a picture task. They were assessed for stuttering behaviors, including:

Primary Behaviors
(i) **Verbal** which includes: Repetition of a part word/full word, Prolongation, Hesitation, Stress, Starters, Blocks etc.

Secondary behaviors
(ii) **Hidden**: Situational fear, Blocks, Struggle or Forcing, Avoidance of words/searching for words.
(iii) **Nonverbal** (Physical concomitants, Facial expression, Gestures, Eye blinking, Gasping)

Other concomitants
   (iv)   Phonology
   (v)   Articulation

Speech analysis: The probands were grouped as mild, moderate or severe CWS based on their score with respect to the instances of: speech repetition, blocks, prolongations and hesitations observed during the performance of the speech and reading tasks. If there was less than a score of 20 it was diagnosed as mild stuttering, moderate if 21 to 50 and severe if more than 50 instances of repetition, prolongations, blocks and hesitations occurred in a given task.

To understand the effect of stuttering on the social behavior of the proband, their academic and extracurricular performance was evaluated with the help of the class teacher. Associated symptoms like embarrassment and anxiety were also discussed. About 85.7% of students who were referred by the teachers were confirmed to be stuttering. CWS identified in this manner were further verified by speech pathologists using video samples to score for primary and secondary behaviors. However, in some schools, videotaping was not possible and, in such instances, we had to depend on audio, along with manual scoring for the secondary behaviors.

3.1.3   Risk factors

The parents of the probands were personally contacted by the investigators in their homes. With their consent a structured interview was conducted to collect information on important risk factors for stuttering that included: pre- and perinatal life; type of dysfluency; physical and emotional stress; handedness; the nature and age at onset of stuttering; parental marriage type, i.e. consanguinity; family history; family attitudes, including information on how they coped with the stuttering in daily life, their awareness of management/treatment; and personal reactions, e.g. anxiety, shyness. A standard set of questions were used to elicit this information (Appendix 4).

3.1.4 Pedigree drawing

Pedigrees were drawn to depict consanguinity and included information on first degree (children, parents and siblings), second degree (grandparents, uncles, aunts, nieces and nephews) and third degree (cousins) relatives wherever available. Other affected members in the family of each proband beyond the nuclear family were not personally assessed due to their unavailability or time constraints. However, additional affected members of the extended family and their persistent/recovery status were recorded, after thorough probing and confirmation by parents and other informants in the family. Nevertheless, it is possible that recovery status was under-reported.

3.2 HOSPITAL DATA

We approached the speech therapy departments of four major hospitals in Chennai. Generally, speech therapy sessions last for prolonged duration; hence Person Who Stutter (PWS) most often being college students, prefer vacation time for the therapy. The self-support group meetings also helped us to collect this data. With prior permission from these hospitals, we ascertained PWS from speech therapy departments and utilized their case histories (Appendix-5).

3.3 INCLUSION CRITERIA: Children with greater than 4% dysfluency (≥ 20 instances) were included for this study.

3.4 EXCLUSION CRITERIA: Although 542 probands were ascertained from schools and hospitals, 60 of them were excluded from the study due to factors like: pre/post-stuttering epilepsy, cleft palate, ADHD, polio, deafness, head injury or onset within six months of our assessment. In the remaining 482 probands ascertained 102 had to be dropped off due to non-participation in the study. Remaining 380 probands formed the study cohort. Further the study cohort was separated into two subgroups as detailed below:

Group I constituted of children with stuttering ascertained from schools. While a total of 303 CWS were ascertained during the first phase of screening, only **180 probands** could be reached out at their homes to meet the parents for further information and detailed pedigree data. In other words, 59% of the parents cooperated for the detailed investigation.

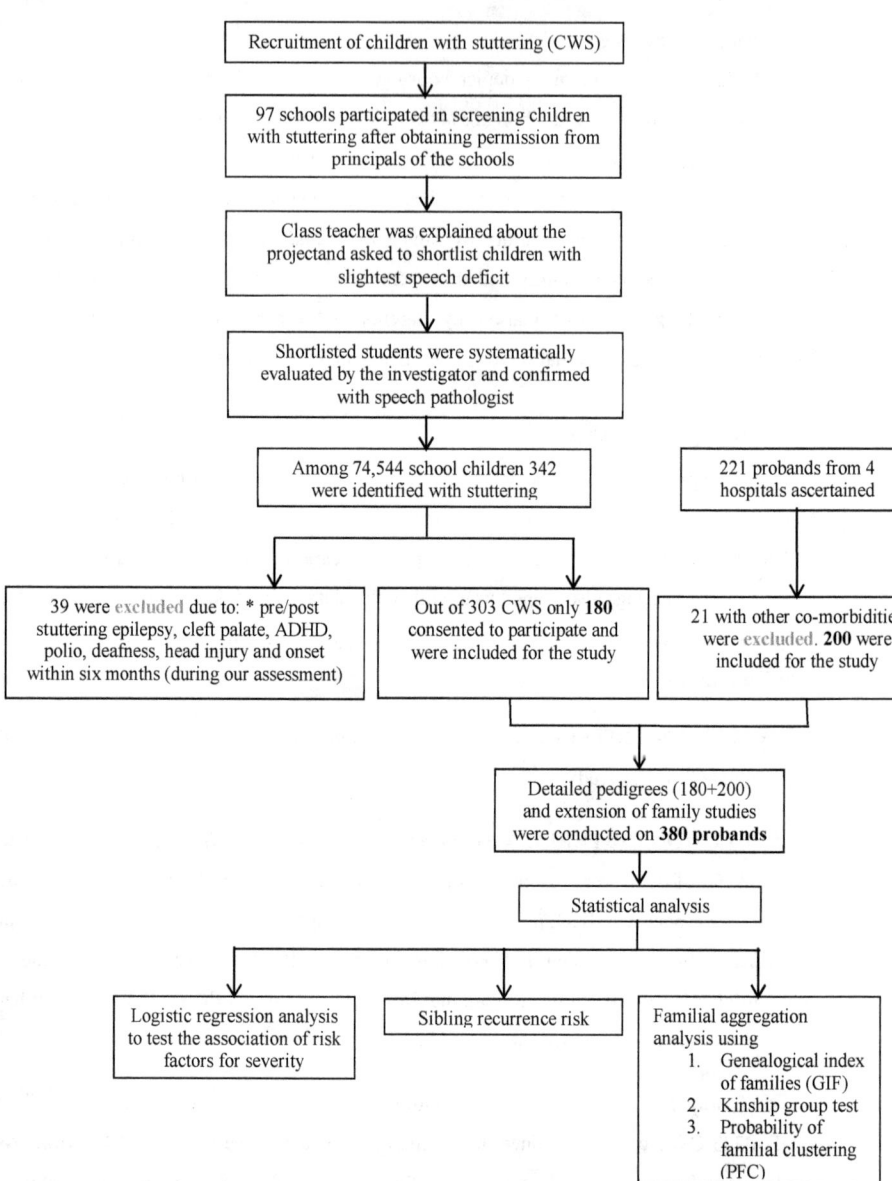

Figure 9: Flow chart depicting the study design and recruitment of 342 children with stuttering used for epidemiological study in phase I

Group II constituted of a mixed age range of persons with stuttering (PWS) essentially ascertained from hospitals. While 221 probands were ascertained only **200 PWS** could be included for the study after applying the exclusion criteria.

Stuttering is indeed complex disorder and diverse, owing to a number of elements involved in depicting stuttering as a phenotype. Given this situation the study design relies on the fact that only when the trait is characterized using different tools we arrive at the severity. So the rationale was to include any individual with stuttering irrespective of the gradient.

3.5 STATISTICAL ANALYSIS

To avoid ascertainment bias, the two groups were subjected to statistical analysis separately. Figure 9 represents the study design of and recruitment of probands in the form of a flow chart in phase I.

3.5.1 Coefficient of inbreeding

The progeny of consanguineous parents is by definition inbred. Consanguinity is measured by the coefficient of inbreeding (F) which is the probability that an individual receives at a given locus two genes that are identical by descent. Coefficients of inbreeding were calculated for the common types of consanguineous matings: uncle-niece, $F = 1/8$; first cousin, $F = 1/16$; first cousin once removed, $F = 1/32$; second cousin, $F = 1/64$; second cousin once removed, $F = 1/128$; and beyond second cousin, $F<1/256$ (Robert *et al.*, 2007). The mean coefficient of inbreeding (α) was estimated for the population using $\alpha = \Sigma PiFi$; where Pi is the proportion of a certain type of consanguineous marriage and Fi is the coefficient of inbreeding of that specific type of consanguineous marriage.

3.5.2 Familial aggregation

The sibling recurrence risk, i.e. the probability of being affected if a sibling is affected was calculated, correcting for single ascertainment bias (Olson & Cordell, 2000). The sibling recurrence risk ratio is defined as $\lambda_s = K_s/p$, where K_s is denoted as the proportion of affected siblings among all siblings of affected persons in a population, and p is the population prevalence of stuttering. The association of risk factors for severity of stuttering was examined using logistic regression (glm function in R) and proportional odds logistic regression (polr function in R package MASS) models.

Familial aggregation was examined using the genealogical index of families (GIF), kinship group, and probability of familial clustering (PFC) tests as implemented in the R package FamAgg. The GIF is the average kinship coefficient K_F, i.e. the probability that two alleles drawn at random from two individuals are identical, between all possible pairs of affected individuals multiplied by 10^5. The p-values were obtained by creating a null distribution of matched unaffected pairs. We used 1000 simulations to generate the statistics under the null distribution. The kinship group test identifies kinship coefficient-based clusters of closely related affected individuals (Johannes et al., 2016), and its significance is evaluated using the null distribution based on random sampling of individuals. The FamAgg package also provides a calculation of PFC using the function implemented in the R package gap (Zhao, 2007). The PFC is calculated using multinomial distribution of affected cases within families (Yu & Zelterman, 2002). Due to the high computational burden for this procedure, the analysis was restricted to pedigrees with fewer than 22 individuals. All of the statistical analyses were performed using the R package (R Core Team, 2016).

PHASE II - MOLECULAR GENETIC ANALYSIS

From the database thus built during the genetic epidemiology study in phase I, a molecular genetics study was taken up as phase II. Separate ethical clearance was obtained in order to continue with the molecular genetic analysis (Approval No: UM/IHEC/10-2017 -I) (Appendix-6).

3.6 PROBAND RECRUITMENT

Since the study lasted for five years many of the students identified initially have migrated to different schools while some did not cooperate. Further the cost factor was another constraint. From the database built in phase I, **64** unrelated probands with non-syndromic persistent stuttering were randomly selected for the mutational analysis. The ancestry of the probands was determined by self-report or from parents and essentially traces back to Tamil Nadu; all probands were Asiatic in origin.

Stuttering assessments and documentation were performed by thorough phenotypic characterization using Stuttering Severity Instrument, 3rd edition SSI-3 with the help of experienced speech pathologist, to obtain the diagnostic severity score for all the 64 probands. Informed consent was obtained from all participants or their parents/guardians if they were minors (Appendix 7).

3.7 MOLECULAR METHODS

Eight milliliters of blood were collected by venipuncture method in EDTA coated vacutainers™ (Beckon and Dickinson, USA) from the probands and their nuclear family members and coded systematically.

Genomic DNA was isolated using Phenol Chloroform Isoamyl alcohol (PCI) procedure (Sambrook & Russell, 2001). The precipitated DNA was purified and dissolved in 1X TE buffer (pH-8). The concentration and purity were determined using Nano drop (Thermo- Fisher Scientific, Wilmington, USA), the integrity was checked in 0.8% agarose gel (SeaKem® LE agarose and 1X TBE) and stored at -20ºC.

3.8 MUTATIONAL ANALYSIS OF *GNPTAB*, *GNPTG* AND *NAGPA* GENE MUTATIONS

The 12 specific exons spanning across the three genes viz., *GNPTAB*, *GNPTG*, and *NAGPA* implicated in stuttering were screened. Our analysis was focused to investigate on the known and any novel variants that occurred in these twelve exons studied. Primer sequences were adapted from Kang *et al.*, 2010, after improvising using NCBI's Primer-BLAST(*Https://WWW.Ncbi.Nlm.Nih.Gov/Tools/Primer-Blast/*, n.d.; Ye *et al.*, 2012) the sequence coverage of exon 10 of the *NAGPA* gene (Table 4). As a cost-effective approach, we selected these 12 exons to observe the recurrence of mutation in our ethnic population that is unexplored to this date.

The amplified PCR products were purified by the FavorPrep™ PCR purification kit (FAVORGEN, Taiwan). The amplicons were sequenced using ABI Prism Big-Dye Terminator 3.1 cycle sequence reaction kit on ABI 3730XL automated sequencer (Applied Biosystems, USA). Chromatograms were analyzed using NCBI nucleotide BLAST

(*Https://Blast.Ncbi.Nlm.Nih.Gov/Blast.Cgi*, n.d.; Johnson *et al.*, 2008) and UCSC genome browser BLAT(*Genome.Ucsc.Edu*, n.d.; Kent *et al.*, 2002) (GRCh37/hg19 build).

Table 4: Primer pairs of *GNPTAB*, *GNPTG* & *NAGPA* used for PCR and DNA sequencing

GENE Exon No	Forward primer (5'-3')	Reverse primer (5'-3')	Annealing Temp (°C)	Product size (bp)
GNPTAB				
9	TGCTGTCTCTTTGAATTTTGG	AGGAAGGGAAGGCAATGAAG	60	521
11	TCAACGCAGCAGGATCTAAA	AGGTTTGCACCACCACACTT	61	591
13_1	CAAGGACGACATGCAAATTC	GCGTCTTTTGGAAGGAGTGA	61	649
13_2	TACAGCCCAGAAGGGTTACG	AATCAGAGATGGGGGCTTTT	62	597
13_3	TGCAGAGGTTGACTTTTCCTG	TCACACTTGGGCTGTTTCCT	62	597
19	TCATTCCCCCAGAGAATCAT	AGCTTGGGCAACAAGAACAA	60	460
GNPTG				
1	AGGCCCTCAAACCCTGAC	TCCTCCACCACCTTCATCTT	62	497
2	GTTGCTCCTCGGGCTCTC	AAGGCTGACAAACCAATGCT	62	435
9 & 10	CAGGACCTGGCCGATGAG	AGTTTCTGCCAAAACACCAG	62	500
NAGPA				
Exon 2	TCCTCTGGGAAGCGTCCGG	GTTAAGTGACTTGAACACGG	62	677
Exon 6&7	GGGCAGCCTGGAGGGAGTT	GAGACAGAAGCAGCAGAGGA	62	489
Exon 10	TCTTAAATGTTGCCCCATCC	CAGCGGAGCATGGTATTGCTA	59	594

Variants identified were predicted using VarSome (*Https://Varsome.Com*, n.d.; Kopanos *et al.*, 2019) tools include various predictors like DANN, Mutation taster, Likelihood Ratio Test - LRT, Mutation Assessor, SIFT, Provean, etc.,) and Polyphen tool, to deduce the pathogenicity. It was classified according to ACMG guidelines along with the ACMG attributes. The guidelines describe the process of classifying variants into five categories as "pathogenic," "likely pathogenic," "uncertain significance," "likely benign," and "benign", based on the evidence from computational data, population data, functional data, segregation data (Richards *et al.*, 2015). Cosegregation of the pathogenic variants among the family members was also evaluated. The novelty and frequency of the variants were compared with the gnomAD database that served as a control. They represent the general population and few individuals may likely be affected or recovered from the disorder of interest.

Effects of p. Glu1200Lys and p. Iso268Leu amino acid change in GNPTAB and GNPTG protein respectively

Both the native and mutated protein of GNPTAB and GNPTG were subjected to pair-wise alignment using the Geneious Pro version 6.1.2 (*Http://Www.Geneious.Com/Download.*, n.d.; Katoh K, 2013). The pair-wise alignment was carried out by MAFFT alignment. Default parameters were set to assess and predict the effect of SNP identified in this study.

Impact of a *de novo* variant c.802A>C/+ (p. Ile268Leu) by quantifying gene expression

To study the impact of a *de novo* heterozygous variant (**c.802A>C/+**) in *GNPTG* gene identified in one family (STU 63), mRNA expression profile, and lysosomal enzyme study was performed along with mucolipidosis screening test. The proband was the only individual affected with stuttering, while his father, mother, and sister served as normal speaking controls. The plasma collected from fresh blood (5 ml) was used to study the enzyme activity. RNA was isolated using mirVana miRNA isolation kit (Invitrogen, USA) as per the manufacturer's protocol and checked for integrity and purity (Figure 10).

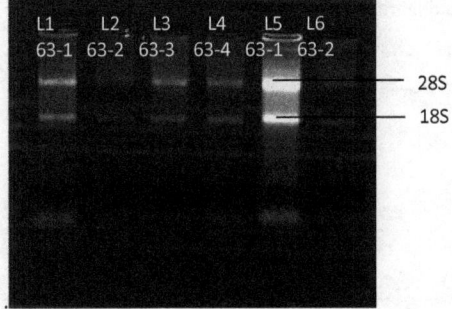

Figure 10: RNA integrity analysis by agarose gel electrophoresis. The 28S and 18S rRNA bands are indicated. The lanes L1-4 represents four samples and L5-6 are duplicates with different dilution

A two-step qRT-PCR was used to measure the transcript levels of the mRNAs of interest.

1. From 500ng of total RNA, cDNA was synthesized using the RevertAid First Strand cDNA Synthesis Kit (Thermo Scientific, USA) according to the manufacturer's instruction in ABI GeneAmp 9700 PCR System. A reverse transcription reaction mix of 20µl was prepared and was loaded on to ABI GeneAmp 9700 PCR System
2. For quantifying gene expression real-time Quantitative PCR was performed on QuantStudio3 Real-Time PCR System using GoTaq DNA polymerase (Promega) in the presence of SYBR Green. The primers specific for the transcripts of *GNPTAB, GNPTG,* and *NAGPA* (**Table 5**) were designed with the aid of IDT software (*Https://Sg.Idtdna.Com/*, n.d.; Owczarzy *et al.,* 2008) and checked for specificity with NCBI's primer-blast. The annealing temperature of the primers was optimized using temperature gradient PCR. Reaction mix for the samples under investigation along with NTC (no template control) was prepared in triplicates for *GNPTAB, GNPTG, NAGPA,* and *ACTB* genes. The reaction mix was loaded onto a 96 well plate and sealed with MicroAmp® Optical Adhesive Film (Applied Biosystems).

Ct value (cycle threshold) is the number of PCR cycles required to achieve a given level of fluorescence. Since the Ct value is proportional to the logarithm of the initial amount of the target, the relative concentration of one target with another is reflected as a difference in cycle number (ΔCt) that is necessary to achieve an equivalent level of fluorescence. The expression levels of *GNPTAB, GNPTG,* and *NAGPA* were measured by relative quantification using the ΔCt method with β-actin gene *ACTB* as endogenous control (Melt curve plot: Figure 11).

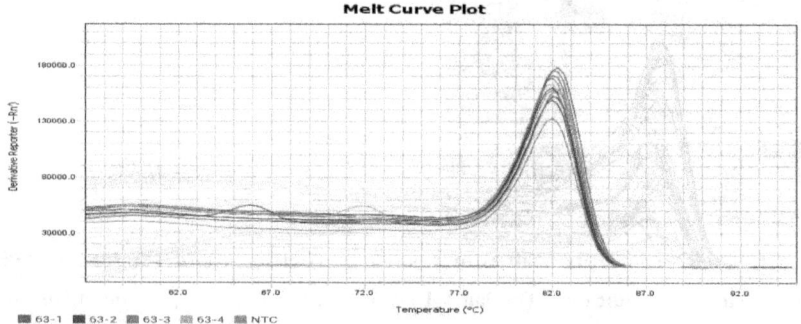

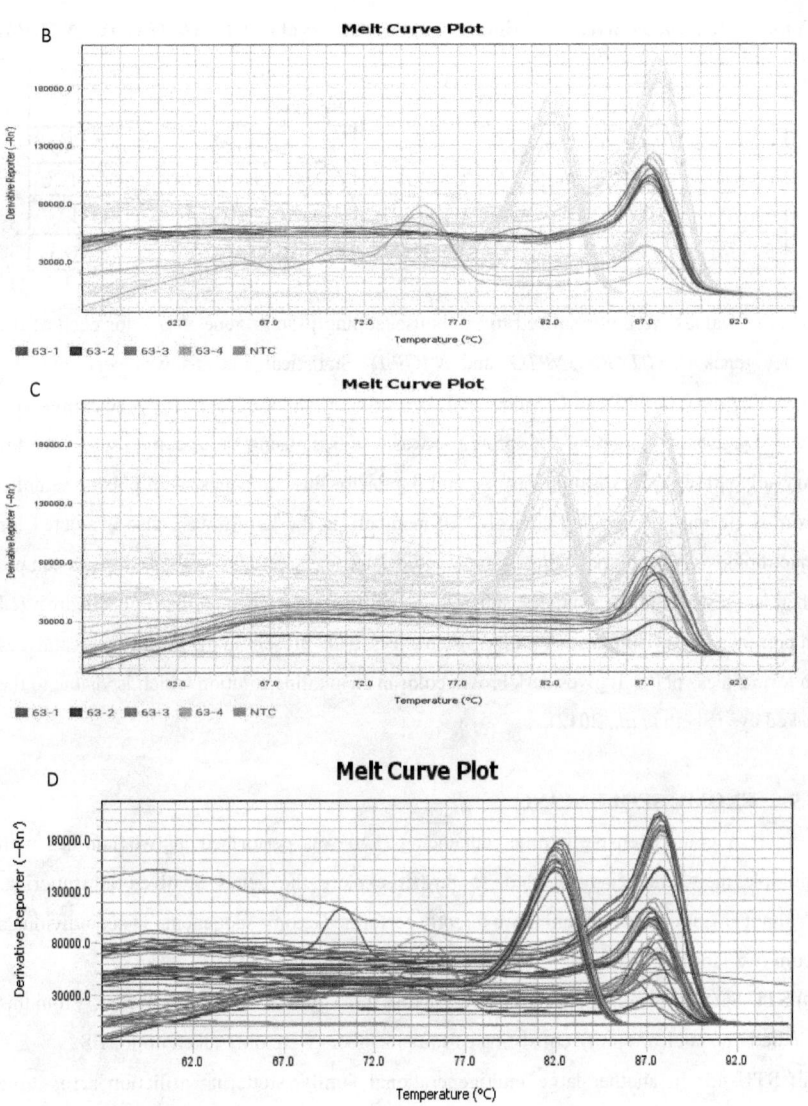

Figure 11: Melt curve plot from qPCR of (A) *GNPTAB* (B) *GNPTG* (C) *NAGPA* (D) All three genes along with β-actin control gene

Table 5: Real time nucleotide primer sequences of target (*GNPTAB*, *GNPTG*, *NAGPA*) and endogenous (*β-actin*) genes

GENE	Forward primer (5'-3')	Reverse primer (5'-3')
GNPTAB	TGGCTCGCTGATAAGTTCTG	GTGAGTCTGGTTTGGGAGAAG
GNPTG	CCTTGCTAGTGTACCCAACC	GGTCTTTAAGTAGCCAGCATCC
NAGPA	CTCCAGAGTAAAGCAGTGTCTC	AGGAGCAAGGACAGGTTTG
β-actin	ACCTTCTACAATGAGCTGCG	CCTGGATAGCAACGTACATGG

Delta Ct values were normalized to the housekeeping β-actin gene *ACTB* for each of the target genes (*GNPTAB*, *GNPTG*, and *NAGPA*). Statistical analysis was performed by averaging the control Delta Ct values and comparing it with the respective gene expression.

Lysosomal targeting of proteins was studied using a specific substrate for Arylsulphatase A, Hexosaminidase A, and β galactosidase enzymes, with plasma samples from stuttering proband and controls. All members in the family were also evaluated for mucolipidosis phenotype using a rapid colorimetric screening method. It is a simple chemical test where the synthetic substrate pNCS (p-nitrocatechol sulfate) gets hydrolyzed in presence of Arylsulfatase-A (ASA) when excessively present in the plasma and catalyzes to form excess pNC. It gives dark brown color in an alkaline solution which is visible to the naked eye (Sheth *et al.*, 2012).

3.9 EXOME SEQUENCING

A comprehensive exome sequencing (ES) was performed in two families with multiple members being affected, to further explore the genes involved in stuttering. Without any prior gene screening we directly performed exome sequencing in six individuals from two families.

(i) **STU 66:** In this family seven members across three generations were affected. From this kindred one nuclear family consisting of **four** members were only taken up for ES.

(ii) **STU 65:** In another large multigenerational family, stuttering affliction across five generations were documented based on detailed pedigree. From this family, **two** affected siblings born to affected consanguineous parents, were taken up for ES.

ES was commercially carried out at MedGenome Labs Ltd., Bangalore facility as described below. The exome sequencing library was prepared using Agilent-Sure Select XT Reagent Kit (Illumina). Biotinylated oligonucleotide capture probes (V5+UTR) designed for all the coding exons were used to enrich the region of interest (exome) by hybridization. The DNA was sheared and the adapter sequence was added to those DNA fragments and paired-end libraries were generated. The resulting adaptor-ligated library was hybridized with exome-specific biotinylated capture library. The target molecules are then enriched using streptavidin beads followed by amplification. At each step the products were purified using AMPure beads and quantified.

The library obtained was diluted to final concentration of 2nm in 10ul and subjected to Cluster amplification. The flow cell was loaded on to the sequencer (Hi Seq X10) to generate 2X150 bp sequence reads at 100x sequencing depth. Sequenced data with Q30 values was considered as qualified and processed to generate FASTQ files for further downstream variant analysis (Figure 12).

The raw data was then quality trimmed and reads (using fastq-mcf command line tool) were aligned to Human Reference genome (hg19) (Build - GrCh37, obtained from https://genome.ucsc.edu/) using BWA-MEM. The output in SAM format is converted to BAM file (using Samtools) and processed to obtain SNVs (Single Nucleotide Variation) and INDELs (small insertions and deletions) in a standard VCF (Variant call format) file. Coverage of the genes were analyzed using Bedtools.

The variants were called using GATK software and annotated using MedGenome in-house variant annotation pipeline (VariMAT - Variation and Mutation Annotation Toolkit). It integrates multiple clinical grade databases (GWAS, ClinVar, OMIM, SwissVar, ExAC, dbSNP, 1000 genomes), variant class prediction and variants pathogenicity prediction tools for annotating the variants. VariMAT annotated variants contain information on the population frequency, computational pathogenicity prediction, variant type and predicted impact of the variant on the protein (missense, loss of function, etc.) (Figure 13).

Downstream variant analysis

The downstream variant analysis protocol involves short listing of the variants in the affected individuals, followed by prioritization of variants based on the data from additional family members. The huge set of filtered variants were sequentially filtered by primarily using the population specific databases like 1000 genomes, ExAC and GnomAD. Further, emphasis was given to high impact (Frameshift and splice site mutations), moderate impact (missense, indels and silent splice site proximal variations) followed by UTR variants. With no adequate molecular genetics study in stuttering, this study also pays close attention to the novel candidate and known gene variants for their role in stuttering.

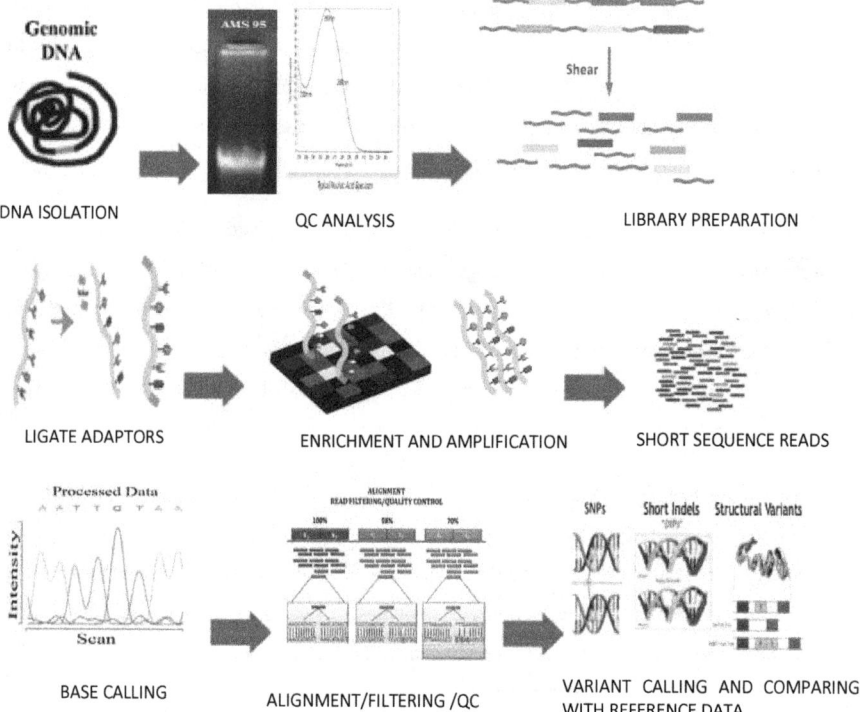

Figure 12: Schematic representation of the ES workflow

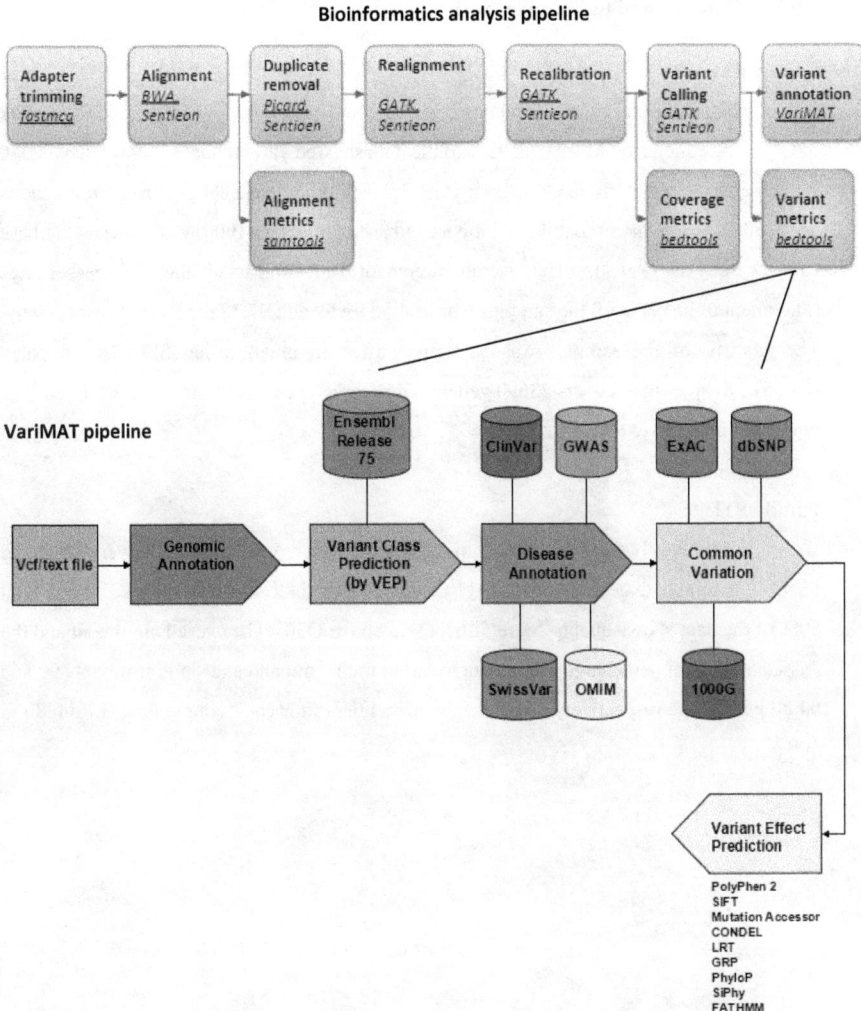

Figure 13: Bioinformatics analysis pipeline (adapted from MedGenome's protocol)

3.9.1 Exome data of two families with stuttering

Family STU 66

The paired-end exome sequencing, generated a data of 10-14 Gb for each of the four individuals sequenced. More than 93% of the data showed variant quality scores above Q30 (Q score measures the base calling accuracy by estimating base calling error probabilities and Q30 indicates the probability of incorrect base call of 1 in 1000 which means the base call accuracy is 99.9%). The overall alignment and the passed alignment percentage (alignment to hg19) in all the samples was around 99.99 and 97.28 percentage respectively. The analysis of the samples was performed after alignment using SS-V5-UTR panel (74,557,381bp) which covers 23690 genes. The average panel depth for each of the sample ranged from 80.42 to 99.27X.

Family STU 65

In this family the proband and his affected brother, V-33 and V-35, were subjected for ES; the total data generated was 8-11 Gb for both the individuals sequenced. More than 90% of the data shows quality score distribution above Q30. The overall alignment and the passed alignment percentage (alignment to hg19) in the proband and sib is around 99.99 and 94.89 percentage respectively. The average panel depth for each sample ranges from 80 to 100 X.

CHAPTER 4
RESULTS

GENETIC EPIDEMIOLOGY

4.1 PREVALENCE OF STUTTERING

We screened 74,544 children in the age group 2.5–16 years and found a prevalence of 0.46% stuttering (N=342 CWS) (95% CI=0.41% - 0.51%).

4.2 RISK FACTORS

Developmental stuttering is a complex phenotype with overt symptomology accompanied by secondary behaviours. Adding to the complexity 80% of the childhood stuttering recover naturally. Despite strong genetic component deterministic risk factors in the form of gender, age at onset, family history, consanguinity, birth order and distribution of sibship size, caste endogamy, attitude etc., contribute additional challenges in understanding the phenotypic variance in stuttering. The following sections will present each factor in detail for both the school and hospital data. It is not permissible to amalgamate the data derived from schools, where the primary diagnosis is by a teacher, with those cases recruited from a hospital where: i) the child has been presumably first referred for specialist advice, and ii) the diagnosis is by a person with relevant diagnostic experience. Also, the hospital-based study sample might be more severely affected and/or may be the families of the school-based sample be less economically secure. The possibility to use all of the cases to study possible inter-relationships between stuttering and the variables under study is not recommended.

4.2.1 Sex ratio

The sex ratio is the ratio of males to females in a population. In most sexually reproducing species, the ratio tends to be 1:1. The male/female sex ratio within the probands was 6:1 (Table 6). The sex ratio by age groups shows an increase from younger to older age groups (Table 7). Among relatives of female probands it was 2:1 and that of male probands it was 4:1 (Table 8). For affected first-degree relatives the sex ratios varied:

female probands had more affected female relatives (M/F = 0.5) while male probands had a higher proportion of affected male relatives (M/F=2:1).

The sex ratio observed in the hospital data was 7:1. Sex ratio by age groups shows a similar trend as school, which increases from younger to older age groups. The sex ratio among relatives of male and female probands are 5:1 and 4:1 respectively which is pronouncedly on the high. Among relatives of female and male probands it was 4:1.

Table 6: Comparison of sex ratio (familial Vs sporadic) among person with stuttering

SEX	POSITIVE FAMILY HISTORY			NEGATIVE FAMILY HISTORY			TOTAL
	SCHOOL	HOSPITAL	TOTAL	SCHOOL	HOSPITAL	TOTAL	
M	86	93	179 (86%)	68	83	151(88%)	330
F	15	14	29 (14%)	11	10	21(12%)	50
TOTAL	101	107	208 (54.7%)	79	93	172 (45.3%)	380
M/F	6:1	7:1	6:1	6:1	8:1	7:1	7:1

Table 7: Frequency distribution of person with stuttering in relation to age and sex ratios

Age (Yrs)	SCHOOL				HOSPITAL			
	M	F	Total	M/F	M	F	Total	M/F
2-5	5	3	8	1.6	5	3	8	1.6
6-10	32	14	46	2	26	7	33	3.7
11-15	92	10	102	9	32	8	40	4
16-20	24	-	24	24	35	4	39	8.8
21-25					39	2	41	19.5
26-30					21		21	
31-35					6		6	
35-40					7		7	
40-45					3		3	
46-50					-			
51-55					1		1	
56-60					1		1	
Total	153	27	180		176	24	200	

Determining recovery is challenging and often requires follow up over time, in our study we have recorded the recovery status retrospectively from informants. In most cases the information on recovery was given by the parents of the proband. Wherever possible, close associates living along with the family such as the grandparents substantiated the information. The recovery rates recorded among the families of male and female probands were 23% and 38% respectively.

Table 8: Frequency of stuttering among the relatives of male and female probands

PROBANDS	AFFECTED MALE RELATIVES/TOTAL MALE RELATIVES			AFFECTED FEMALE RELATIVES/TOTAL FEMALE RELATIVES			M/F	TOTAL AFFECTED RELATIVES/ TOTAL RELATIVES
	SCHOOL	HOSPITAL	TOTAL	SCHOOL	HOSPITAL	TOTAL		
MALE (179)	123/690 =0.18	117/827 =0.14	240/1517 =0.16	34/675 =0.05	26/777 =0.03	60/1452 =0.04	4:1	300/2969 =0.10
FEMALE (29)	16/123 =0.13	23/142 =0.16	39/265 =0.15	10/108 =0.09	6/144 =0.04	16/252 =0.06	2:1	55/514 =0.10
Total (380)	139/813= 0.17	140/969 =0.14	279/1782 =0.16	44/783=0.05	32/921= 0.03	76/1704 =0.04	4:1	355/3486 =0.10

4.2.2 Age at onset

The mean age at onset of stuttering among all the probands was 4.7 years (SD=2.51). The difference in the mean age of onset between males (Mean = 4.8; SD=2.585) and females (Mean = 4.0; SD=1.936) was not significant (t=1.648; P=0.108). Majority (76.6%) of CWS were dysfluent at <6 years and 15.6% at >6 years. The age of onset was not known for 7.8% of the study sample. The frequency of the age of onset among males and females showed two peaks at the $3^{rd.}$ and $5^{th.}$ years respectively. The **manner of onset** was gradual for 71.6% of probands and sudden for 27.2% (Table 9).

The mean **age at onset** was 4.73 (SD=2.68) among probands from hospital which is similar to that of school data. Nearly one fourth (22.5%) in this cohort were not able to specify the manner of onset as opposed to school data (1%). This may be due to their inability to recollect owing to the long-time gap involved. In both the data sets the manner of onset was predominantly gradual.

Table 9: Manner of onset among stuttering probands

PROBANDS	GRADUAL					SUDDEN					
	SCHOOL		HOSPITAL		TOTAL	SCHOOL		HOSPITAL		TOTAL	NK
	FAMILIAL	SPORADIC	FAMILIAL	SPORADIC		FAMILIAL	SPORADIC	FAMILIAL	SPORADIC		
MALE	65	46	43	51	205	20	21	24	16	81	44
FEMALE	12	6	10	4	32	3	5	3	4	15	3
TOTAL	77	52	53	55	237	23	26	27	20	96	47

Table 10: Frequency of stuttering among first-, second- and third-degree relatives of probands with a positive family history

PROBANDS	FIRST DEGREE RELATIVES							SECOND DEGREE RELATIVES							THIRD DEGREE RELATIVES						
	SCHOOL		HOSPITAL		TOTAL		T	SCHOOL		HOSPITAL		TOTAL		T	SCHOOL		HOSPITAL		TOTAL		T
	M	F	M	F	M	F		M	F	M	F	M	F		M	F	M	F	M	F	
MALE	43/165 =0.26	14/146 =0.1	49/177 =0.3	13/175 =0.1	92/342 =0.27	27/321 =0.08	119/663 =0.18	43/394 =0.11	14/407 =0.03	28/415 =0.08	8/388 =0.02	71/809 =0.1	22/795 =0.03	93/1604 =0.06	37/131 =0.28	6/122 =0.05	42/248 =0.2	9/223 =0.04	79/379 =0.21	12/305 =0.04	91/684 =0.13
FEMALE	4/23 =0.17	7/31 =0.23	7/22 =0.3	4/21 =0.2	11/45 =0.24	11/52 =0.21	22/97 =0.23	9/77 =0.12	1/62 =0.02	8/65 =0.1	0/77 =0	17/142 =0.12	1/139 =0.01	18/281 =0.06	3/23 =0.13	2/15 0.13	7/55 =0.1	2/46 =0.04	10/78 =0.13	4/61 =0.1	14/139 =0.1
TOTAL	47/188 =0.25	21/177 =0.12	56/199 =0.3	17/196 =0.1	103/387 =0.27	38/373 =0.1	141/760 =0.19	52/471 =0.11	15/469 =0.03	36/480 =0.08	8/465 =0.02	88/951 =0.1	23/934 =0.02	111/1885 =0.06	40/154 =0.26	8/137 =0.06	49/303 =0.2	11/269 =0.04	89/457 =0.2	19/406 =0.05	108/863 =0.13

4.2.3 Familial data

On analyzing the pedigrees, 56% had a positive family history (n=101/180) and the remaining (n = 79) were sporadic, with a single affected in the family among school and 53.5% (107/200) among hospital data. Similarly, the distribution of affected members among first-, second- and third-degree relatives were 38.2% (68/178), 34.8% (62/178) and 26.9% (48/178) respectively for school and 41.2% (73/177), 24.9% (44/177) and 33.9% (60/177) respectively for hospital. The familial incidence was 11% (178 were stuttering relatives out of 1596 relatives ascertained); 38% of whom were first degree relatives (n = 68) of the probands. The proportion of male stuttering relatives (0.17) was significantly higher than that of female stuttering relatives (0.05) (z=7.6144; P=0.00) (Table 10). The familial incidence was found to be 9% (177/1912) for the hospital data.

4.2.4 Consanguinity

CWS born to non-consanguineous (78%) and consanguineous (22%) parents are shown in Table 11. Among 79 sporadic cases, 11 had consanguineous parents. However, as expected parental consanguinity was higher (71.8%) in familial cases than in sporadic (28.2%). The overall coefficient of inbreeding (α) was 0.0165 (Table 12). Stuttering probands were distributed across the different religions (Table 13). The coefficient of inbreeding (α) for Hindus was 0.0137, 0.0207 for Christians and 0.0088 for Muslims (Table A2).

Among hospital data probands born to consanguineous parents were found to be 23.5%. Consanguinity is a determining factor in both familial (53.3%) and sporadic cases (46.8%) suggesting for an increased role for genetic factors, in stuttering, among the hospital data. The overall coefficient of inbreeding was found to be 0.0110. Although probands were majorly from Hindu religion (74%), recording of religion was unavailable for 23.5%. The religion wise inbreeding coefficient is given (Table A3).

Table 11: Distribution of parental consanguinity among sporadic and familial stuttering probands

Group	School data			Hospital data		
	Sporadic	Familial	Total	Sporadic	Familial	Total
Consanguineous	11 (28.2%)	28 (71.8%)	39 (22%)	22 (46.8%)	25 (53.2%)	47 (23.5%)
Non consanguineous	68 (48.2%)	73 (51.8%)	141 (78%)	71 (46.4%)	82 (53.6%)	153 (76.5%)
Total	79	101	180	93	107	200

Table 12: Frequency of parental consanguinity and the coefficient of inbreeding among stuttering probands

Nature of relationship	School					Hospital				
	M	F	Total 180	%	Inbreeding coefficient (f)	M	F	Total 200	%	Inbreeding coefficient (f)
Non-Consanguineou	126	1	141	78		131	22	153		
Consanguineou	29	1	39	22		44	3	47		
Uncle niece	6	5	11	6.	0.0083	10	-	10	5	0.0063
Aunt-nephew	1	-	1	6		-	-	-		
First cousin	17	4	21	11	0.0073	6	1	7	3.5	0.0022
First cousin	3	1	4	2.	0.0007	2	-	2	1	0.0003
Second cousin	2		2	1.	0.0002	26	2	28	14	0.0022
Mean co-efficient of inbreeding (α)					0.0165					0.0110

Table 13: Frequency of parental consanguinity in stuttering probands by religion

RELIGION	SCHOOL			HOSPITAL		
	CONSANGUINEOUS	NON CONSANGUINEOUS	TOTAL	CONSANGUINEOUS	NON CONSANGUINEOUS	TOTAL
HINDU	21	95	116	35	113	148
MUSLIM	3	12	15	1	2	3
CHRISTIAN	1	5	6	-	1	1
JAIN	0	2	2	-	-	-
UNSPECIFI	13	20	33	13	34	47
INTERCAST	1	7	8	-	1	1
TOTAL	39	141	180	49	151	200

4.2.5 Birth order and distribution of sibship size helps to determine whether CWS are randomly distributed among the birth ranks: 43.3% were first-born, 33.3% were second, 11.0% were third and 8.3% were fourth-born. The average sibship size was 3.0 (SD=1.0). Approximately one in eleven (8/101) subjects were a "single stuttering child" family (7.9%). The majority of families has a sibship size of two (44.5%), 24.8% had 3 sibs, with the frequency of 4-8 siblings gradually decreasing (Table A4). Similar to school data there is an increase in ratio of males to females in all sibship sizes: 43% (86/200) were first born, 36.5% (73/200) were second and 13% (26/200) third born. This trend is similar in both school and hospital data. Approximately 1 in 12 (8/107) subjects were single stuttering child (7.5%), while 45.8% (49/107) are of sibship size two, 31.8% (34/107) sibship size three and gradually decreases in frequency with increase in sibship size (Table A5).

An increased ratio of males to females was consistently observed in all sibship sizes, including the single affected families. Among the 101 probands with a family history, 60.4% (61 probands) had normal speaking parents. The remaining 38.6% had either one (Affected x Normal=39) or both (Affected x Affected=1) parents affected. Among 107 probands from hospital those with family history 64.5% (69 probands) had normal speaking parents and remaining 35.5% (affected x Normal = 38) had one parent affected.

4.2.6 Caste endogamy

Despite linguistic homogeneity in the study population, the cultural barrier created by *caste endogamy* in the majority Hindu population may prevent gene flow between sub-communities and thus could be a partial contributor to genetic diversification. Only 4.4% of the affected children were born to parents in inter-caste marriages. Thirty-six endogamous castes were recorded among Hindu probands (67.9%), but in 18.3% of cases no specific caste was reported. In addition, probands belonging to Christian (2.2%) and Muslim (7.2%) communities were also recorded (Table A6). Thirty-seven endogamous castes were recorded among Hindu probands in hospital data. In addition, probands belonging to Christian (2%) and Muslim (2.5%) communities were also recorded (TableA7).

4.2.7 Attitude

Speech therapy awareness was conspicuously absent in 84% of probands' families. Attitudinal inhibitions, such as avoidance of speech with strangers, were observed. Coping involved interjections and word substitutions. Stress factors such as prenatal complications, speech delays, multilingual environment in the educational setting, social/parental pressure and illness were attributed as a reason for stuttering in their children. Only 20.5% of the parents discussed such stress factors (Table 14).

Table 14: Stress factors studied among stuttering probands

S.No.	Stress variables	Description
1	Prenatal	Complications during birth, prematurity, etc.
2	Medical	Illness/disease
3	Social	Behavior in class, peer pressure
4	Parental	Parental/sibling pressure
5	Education	Multilingual and advanced language skills
6	Developmental	Milestone delay, especially speech

About 20.5% of our probands reported some kind of these stress variables attributed to their stuttering. The predominant stress factor appears to be prenatal (57.7%) > developmental milestone (22%) > medical (11.5%) > educational (2.6%).

4.3 FAMILIAL AGGREGATION - SCHOOL DATA

The age of onset, sex, family history, and consanguinity were examined for their association with severity of stuttering. The distribution of degree of severity among the probands (n = 180) showed that in 51.6% of cases stuttering was mild, with 22.7% moderate and 25.0% severe. The degree of severity among probands (n = 200) is almost equally distributed in the hospital data while the mild category (51.6%) is high in the school data (Table 15). Severity was grouped into three groups (mild, moderate and severe) and two (mild, moderate versus severe) and tested for its association with risk factors using proportional odds logistic regression and logistic regression models (Table 16&17).

Table 15: Distribution of severity of stuttering among the probands

PROBANDS	School				Hospital			
	MILD	MODERATE	SEVERE	TOTAL	MILD	MODERATE	SEVERE	TOTAL
Familial	55	20	26	101	28	39	40	107
Sporadic	38	21	20	79	32	34	27	93
TOTAL	93	41	45	180	60	73	67	200

There was suggestive evidence for association of age and sex with severity (unadjusted p-value < 0.05) under logistic regression model. However, sex would be the only factor associated with severity, if a conservative Bonferroni multiple-test correction was applied to the p-values, assuming 4 independent tests. As shown in Table 16 the severity among males was significantly higher than in females. The age of onset among the severe form of stuttering was slightly higher compared to cases of mild stuttering. Logistic regression and proportional odds logistic regression gave similar results. In hospital data there was no suggestive evidence for association of sex and age at onset with severity in contrast to school data (Table 17).

Table 16: Risk factors for severity of stuttering for school data

Variable\Severity	Mild	Moderate	Severe	B (SE)*	P*	B (SE)**	P**
Sex							
Male	74	37	44	-1.37(0.56)	0.01	- 1.35(0.55)	0.01
Female	19	4	2				
Family History No	38	19	22	-0.52(0.33)	0.12	- 0.52(0.31)	0.09
Yes	55	22	24				
Consanguinity No	74	32	35	0.64 (0.42)	0.12	0.59(0.38)	0.12
Yes	19	9	11				
Age at onset	4.25(2.1)	5.59(3.0)	4.92(2.72)	0.15(0.07)	0.03	0.10(0.06)	0.07

Note: *B(SE), p-value under logistic regression; **B(SE), p-value under proportional odds logistic regression; Mean(SD) are presented for age at onset. B-denotes the log odds ratio.

Table 17: Risk factors for severity of stuttering for hospital data

Variable\Severity	Mild	Moderate	Severe	B (SE)*	P*	B (SE)**	P**
Sex							
Male	54	64	59	0.70(0.55)	0.21	0.03(0.42)	0.94
Female	6	11	9				
Family History							
No	32	35	28	0.20(0.35)	0.57	0.24 (0.31)	0.42
Yes	28	40	40				
Consanguinity							
No	46	61	47	-0.24 (0.40)	0.53	0.20(0.37)	0.59
Yes	14	14	21				
Age at onset	4.30(2.48)	4.74(2.59)	5.08(2.88)	0.10(0.07)	0.17	0.09(0.06)	0.15

Note: *B(SE), p-value under logistic regression; **B(SE), p-value under proportional odds logistic regression; Mean(SD) are presented for age at onset. B-denotes the log odds ratio.

4.4 FAMILIAL AGGREGATION MEASURES - SCHOOL DATA

4.4.1 Genealogical Index

As expected, the GIF (mean $K_F \times 10^5$) of all pedigrees was 84.60 (p-value = 0.001 based on 1000 simulations) and within consanguineous families (n=39) the GIF was 442.60 (p-value < 0.001), indicating higher kinship among the affected individuals within consanguineous families. The GIF among non-consanguineous pedigrees (n=141) was estimated to be 93.02, which was not statistically significant (p-value=0.127) implying higher kinship among the affected individuals within consanguineous families.

4.4.2 Kinship group test

The kinship group test was used to identify the families with a large proportion of closely related affected individuals. From all the pedigrees examined (n=180) the test identified 14 families (7.8%) which had a higher proportion of closely related affected individuals, of which 5 (5/39=12.8%) were consanguineous families. When applied to consanguineous families the test identified 6 pedigrees (5 families identified in the previous analysis plus additional family) with higher proportion of affected individuals.

4.4.3 Sibling recurrence risk ratio

The sibling recurrence risk (K_s) estimated from the overall sample was 0.143 (SD=0.019), for consanguineous families K_s was 0.11(SD=0.016), and for non-consanguineous families K_s was 0.197 (SD=0.017). The K_s values for consanguineous and non-consanguineous families were significantly different (p-value =0.04). There was a slight increase in the sibling recurrence risk (K_s) estimated within the male sib-pairs 0.17 (SD=0.027) compared to all sib-pairs, but K_s could not be estimated for female sib-pairs pairs since they were not observed in the cohort.

Within the full sample, the sibling recurrence risk ratio $\lambda_s=K_s/p$, assuming 1% prevalence of stuttering, was 14.30 [95% CI= (10.48, 18.12)], and within consanguineous families K_s was 19.68 [95% CI (11.65, 27.72)]. These estimates would double if the prevalence observed in the current sample (~0.5%) was used.

Familial aggregation measures

Familial aggregation measures such as: genealogical index, kinship group test and sibling recurrence risk ratio were calculated separately for hospital data and compared with that of school data. The results show similar trend in both the cohorts in terms of familial aggregation and high sibling recurrence risk ratio among consanguineous families (Table 18)

Table 18: Familial Aggregation indices of both school and hospital data

FAMILIAL AGGREGATION	CATEGORIES	SCHOOL (180)	HOSPITAL (200) C=46 / NC=154	COMBINED FAMILIES
Genealogical Index	All pedigrees	84.60 p-value = 0.001	71.70 p-value = 0.0092	64.560 p-value = 0.0004
	Consanguineous	442.60 p-value < 0.001	368.882 p-value =0.0144	282.58 p-value = 0.0087
	Non Consanguineous	93.02 p-value = 0.127	88.161 p-value=0.064	85.55 p-value=0.001
Kinship group test	All pedigrees	14 (8%)	5(2.5%)	6
	Consanguineous	5 (13%)	6 (13%)	6
Sibling recurrence risk ratio K_s	All pedigrees	0.143 (SD=0.019)	0.16 (SD=0.01)	0.18 (SD=0.007)
	Consanguineous	0.197(SD= 0.041)	0.19(SD=0.02)	0.19(SD=0.014)
	Non Consanguineous	0.11 (SD=0.016)	0.155 (SD=0.011)	0.17 (SD=0.009)

p<0.05 are considered significant

4.5 MOLECULAR GENETIC ANALYSIS OF STUTTERING

This section presents the findings of the three molecular approaches implemented to study individuals with stuttering.

4.5.1 Mutational analysis of the three putative genes in stuttering

A total of 64 unrelated probands with non-syndromic persistent stuttering were randomly selected [sex ratio of 59 males: 5 females (12:1); mean age at onset of 5.13 years] were screened for the recurrence of mutations in the three stuttering implicated genes. Sixty seven percent (43/64) of them had family history. More than 50% of PWS were found to be severe: **53.1% severe** (34/64), **28.1% moderate** (18/64), and **18.8% mild** (12/64).

Mutation screening of the twelve specific exons that were previously reported identified a total of **12 variants** that include five nonsynonymous missense, five synonymous and two non-coding variants (**Tables 19 and 20; Figures A4-A6**). The identified variants and their combinations were analyzed in an Upset plot using R program (*Https://Cran.r-Project.Org/Bin/Windows/Base/*, n.d.; R Core Team, 2016) (**Figure 14**). The plot visualizes intersections of sets as a matrix in which the rows represent variants and the columns represent the number of probands having that particular combination of variants. Thus, each identified variant represents a set and each proband represents an element that is contained in one or more sets. We observed that all the probands had p. Asn495Asn synonymous variant in the *NAGPA* gene in common, along with at least two or more other synonymous variants. Variants like p. Glu1200Lys in *GNPTAB*, 5' UTR (c.-4 C>T), p. Pro234Pro and p. Ile268Leu in *GNPTG* and p. Arg44Pro and p. Leu47Phe in *NAGPA* gene, occurred singly in unrelated probands.

The number of variants observed in *NAGPA* (n=6) was greater than that observed in *GNPTG* (n=4) and *GNPTAB* (n=2) genes. Among the variants identified those missense variants with high conservation scores and pathogenic predictions in both SIFT and Polyphen were examined further in segregation analysis. Three such missense variants, p. Glu1200Lys in

GNPTAB, p. Ile268leu in *GNPTG*, and p. Arg44Pro in *NAGPA* gene, were observed in three unrelated probands.

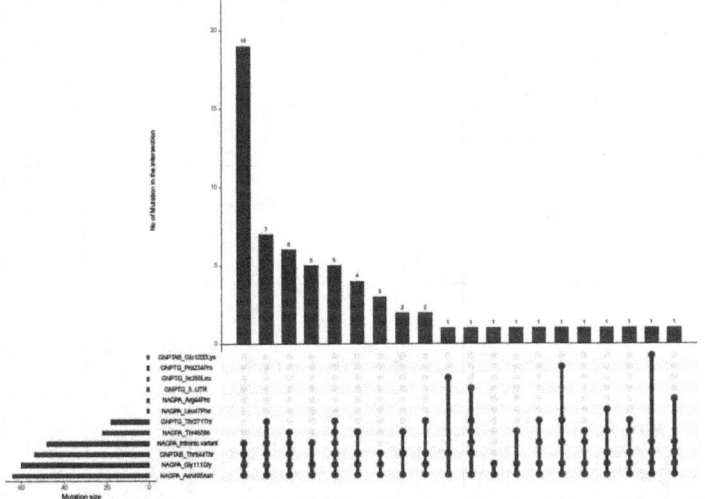

Figure 14: An Upset plot of identified variants in this study across three genes implicated in stuttering to show combination of variants among probands. For each variant that is a part of intersection, a black filled circle is shown in the matrix and for the variant that is not part of intersection, a light gray circle is placed. The number of probands bearing the set of variants (column-based relationships) is emphasized by vertical black line connecting the top most and bottom most black circle. The bar chart on top and left of the matrix gives the size of intersections and sets respectively.

The other two missense variants (p. Leu47Phe & p. Thr465Ile) in *NAGPA*, were observed to have a higher minor allele frequency (MAF) in the gnomAD exome database favoring common variant and likely benign status. Further, these variants showed a low conservation score with benign predictions either in SIFT or Polyphen2. Hence, segregation analysis and genotype-phenotype correlations were performed only for the three missense variants with a high conservation score and low MAF. Though the p. Glu1200Lys variant in the *GNPTAB* gene has high MAF it was still considered for segregation analysis since it has been previously reported (Kang et al., 2010).

Table 19: Allele frequencies of the 12 variants observed in *GNPTAB*, *GNPTG* and *NAGPA* genes among the 64 probands with stuttering and their comparison with gnomAD database

S.No	GENE	Nucleotide change	Amino acid change	Exon	dbSNP ID	Hom/Het (n=64 probands)	Allele frequency (n=128 alleles)	Stuttering studies	Allele frequency in South Asian gnomAD	Allele frequency in total gnomAD
Missense variants										
1	*GNPTAB*	c.3598G>A	p.Glu1200Lys	Exon 19	rs137853825	-/1	0.008	(8/1013) = 0.00789	0.0214	0.0028
2	*GNPTG*	c.802A>C	p.Ile268Leu	Exon 10	rs759796840	-/1	0.008		0.00003266	0.000004
3	*NAGPA*	c.131G>C	p.Arg44pro	Exon 2	rs374266430	-/1	0.008	(1/1013) = 0.000099	0.002851	0.0004
4	*NAGPA*	c.139C>T	p.Leu47Phe	Exon 2	rs371054576	-/1	0.008		0.003873	0.0005
5	*NAGPA*	c.1394 C>T	p.Thr465Ile	Exon 10	rs7188856	-/22	0.172		0.1751	0.2990
Synonymous variants										
6	*GNPTAB*	c.1932A>G	p.Thr644Thr	Exon13	rs10778148	42/12	0.75	120/1708 alleles	0.6236	0.5900
7	*GNPTG*	c.702T>C	p.Pro234Pro	Exon 9	rs532275192	-/1	0.008		0.003560	0.0004
8	*GNPTG*	c.813G>A	p.Thr271Thr	Exon 10	rs377647926	-/18	0.14		unknown	0.00002
9	*NAGPA*	c.333 A>G	p.Gly111Gly	Exon 2	rs2972272	41/19	0.789	229/1708	0.8222	0.6981
10	*NAGPA*	c.1485C>T	p.Asn495Asn	Exon 10	rs887854	42/22	0.828		0.8177	0.6967
Non coding variants										
11	*GNPTG*	-4 C>T	-	5'UTR	rs554707396	-/1	0.008		0.0002703	0.00006
12	*NAGPA*	c.1174+53C>A	-	intron 7	rs2937112	22/26	0.547		Unknown (0.5730 in 1000K)	0.2792

Table 20: Pathogenicity prediction of the variants observed in three genes for stuttering using various bioinformatics tools
DANN score 1: most damaging; D: Damaging; T: Tolerant; PD: Possibly Damaging; B: Benign; VUS: Variant with Uncertain Significance

S.No	Location	Nucleotide change	dbSNP ID	DANN	General	Functional		Conservation			I Mutant v2.0	Consurf Score	VarSome (ACMG guidelines)	Pathogenic assertion	ACMG attributes
					Mutation taster	SIFT	Provean	LRT	Mutation Assessor	PolyPhen-2					
Missense variants															
1	GNPTAB	c.3598G>A	rs137853825	0.9982	Disease causing	D	Damaging	Deleterious	Low	PD	Decreased stability	9	Benign	Benign	BS1, BS2, PP2, PP3, PP5
2	GNPTG	c.802A>C	rs759796840	0.9696	Disease causing	D	Neutral	Deleterious	Medium	PD	Decreased stability	8	Likely Pathogenic	VUS	PS2, PM2, PP2, PP3
3	NAGPA	c.131G>C	rs374266430	0.9819	Polymorphism	D	Damaging	Neutral	Medium	PD	Decreased stability	4	Likely benign	Likely benign	BS1, BP1, BP4
4	NAGPA	c.139C>T	rs371054576	0.8056	Polymorphism	T	Neutral	Neutral	Neutral	B	Decreased stability	1	Likely benign	Likely benign	BS1, BP1, BP4
5	NAGPA	c.1394 C>T	rs7188856	0.3973	Polymorphism automatic	T	Neutral	Neutral	Low	PD	Decreased stability	1	Benign	Benign	BA1, BP1, BP4, BP6
Synonymous variants															
6	GNPTAB	c.1932A>G	rs10778148	0.4236	-	-	-	-	-	-	-	-	Benign	Benign	BA1, BP4, BP6, BP7
7	GNPTG	c.702T>C	rs532275192	0.3353	-	-	-	-	-	-	-	-	Likely benign	Likely benign	PM2, BP4, BP7
8	GNPTG	c.813G>A	rs377647926	0.4781	-	-	-	-	-	-	-	-	VUS	VUS	PM2, BP4
9	NAGPA	c.333 G>A	rs2972272	0.5259	-	-	-	-	-	-	-	-	Benign	Benign	BA1, BP4
10	NAGPA	c.1485C>T	rs8857854	0.7803	-	-	-	-	-	-	-	-	Benign	Benign	BA1, BP4, BP6, BP7
Non coding variants															
11	GNPTG	-4 C>T	rs554707396	0.9074	-	-	-	-	-	-	-	-	VUS	VUS	PM2, BP4
12	NAGPA	c.1174+53C>A	rs2937112	0.7424	-	-	-	-	-	-	-	-	VUS	VUS	PM2, BP4

Chapter 4   *Results*

4.5.2.1. Segregation analysis of families with variants in the three putative stuttering genes
(i)   Family STU 29

The 16 year old proband with stuttering was ascertained from a government boy's higher secondary school in Salem, Tamil Nadu. He was born to non consanguineous parents and had no complications during his birth. His age of onset of stuttering was reported to be 3 years and he was right handed. Severity assessment rated him as severe with excess of prolongations, blocks and difficulties in initial syllables. Secondary behaviours include eye blinking, stiffness of the body, tension in neck and avoidance of eye contact. There was a situational increase in the stuttering such as in a classroom, while speaking with teachers, superiors or opposite sex and when excited/afraid. Both the proband's father and his elder brother had stuttering that could be rated as moderate.

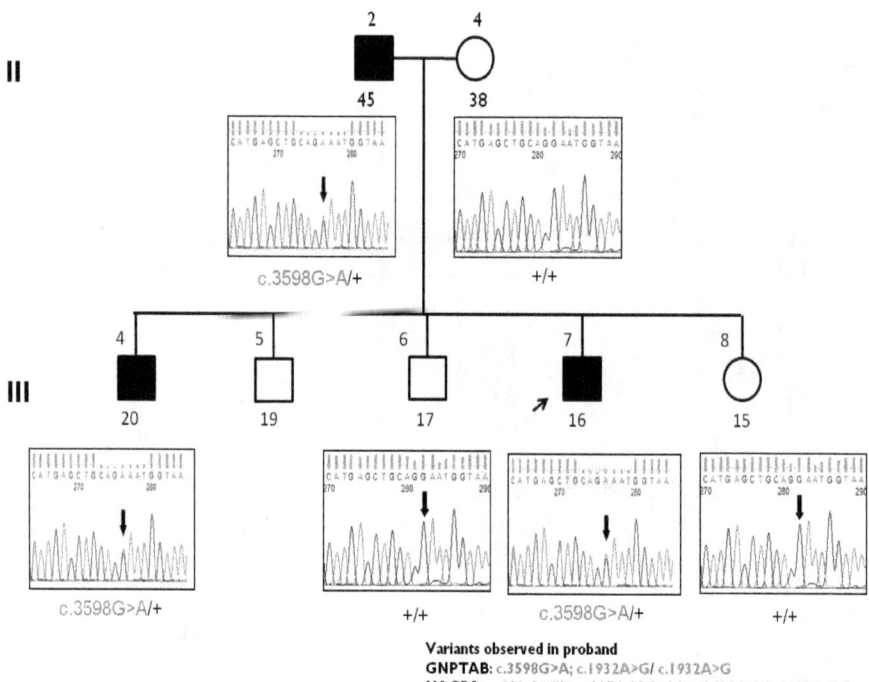

Variants observed in proband
GNPTAB: c.3598G>A; c.1932A>G/ c.1932A>G
NAGPA: c.333 A>G/+; c.1174+53C>A/+;c.1485C>T/c.1485C>T

Figure 15: Partial chromatograms of the Glu1200Lys mutation (*GNPTAB*) segregating in a family with stuttering

Chapter 4 *Results*

Mutational analysis in the proband identified a heterozygous **missense** variant that is in a conserved position p. Glu1200Lys in exon 19 of the *GNPTAB* gene. On extending the analysis to their family members there was cosegregation of the variant with the affected status in a dominant pattern (**Figure 15**).

Furthermore, since this variant was predicted as pathogenic in previous studies it was screened in an additional subset of 26 individuals with severe stuttering. Three of them had this lysine variant resulting in an allele frequency of 2% (4/180), which is similar to that observed in the gnomAD (2.1%). This variant classification according to ACMG is benign (**Table 20**).

(ii) **Family STU 63**

The proband is a 24-year-old male who had normal speech until nine years. Severity assessment rated his stuttering as mild with repetitions, blocks and had eye closure during speech. The proband was born to non-consanguineous parents without any complications during birth. He was right-handed with good academic performance.

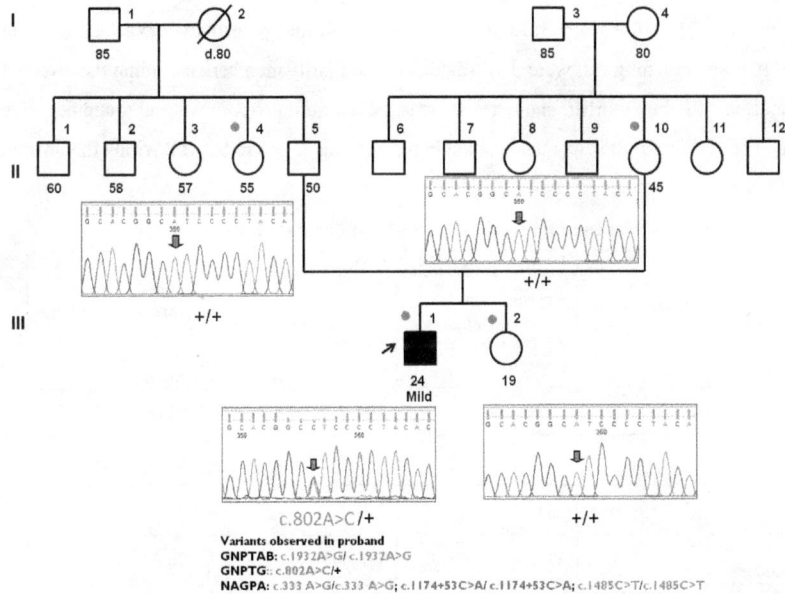

Figure 16: Partial chromatogram of c.802A>C (Ile268Leu) variation in *GNPTG* gene

Mutation analysis of the proband identified a **missense heterozygous missense variant p. Ile268Leu in exon 10 of the *GNPTG* gene**. On extending the analysis to his family members, his unaffected father, mother and sister did not show this variation. Since this is not present in either of the parent but only observed in the proband, it is identified as a *de novo* variant (**Figure 16**). There were no other synonymous variants in the sequenced region to check for the consistency of the paternity. Hence, we typed for Rh blood group phenotype that was found to be consistent with paternity.

As per the ACMG guidelines the variant is classified as "likely pathogenic". Considering the non-consanguineous pedigree, and confirmed *de novo* status of the variant in the affected individual, the variant in *GNPTG* likely favors the gene-disease relationship with a dominant mode of action.

Impact of the *de novo* missense variant (c.802A>C/+ in *GNPTG*)

The importance of heterozygous allele in *GNPTG* gene and its relevance in dysfluency disorder, as opposed to the reported recessive mucolipidosis III phenotype due to homozygous truncation of the same *GNPTG* gene was investigated. To study the impact of this *de novo* heterozygous variant (c.802A>C/+), mRNA expression profile and lysosomal enzyme assay along with mucolipidosis screening test were performed. All the family members including the affected proband, unaffected father, mother, and sister, were screened for mucolipidosis and found negative for the test. The activity of the enzymes studied in plasma was found to be well within the normal range (**Table 21**).

Table 21: Lysosomal enzyme study in the plasma of a stuttering family

Family STU 63	Genotype of *GNPTG* gene	LYSOSOMAL ENZYMES		
		Arylsulfatase A (Normal Range 30–268 nmol/hr/ mg protein)	Hexosaminidase – A (Normal Range 90-385nmol/hr/mg protein)	B- galactosidase (Normal Range 470–2500nmol/hr/mg protein)
STU 63-1 (proband)	c.802A>C/+	32.6	106.9	581.6
STU 63-2 (father) unaffected	+/+	31.9	108.1	489.7
STU 63-3 (mother) unaffected	+/+	38.2	113.1	631.9
STU 63-4 (sister) unaffected	+/+	33.6	116.1	506.3

■ **Likely pathogenic variant**

To quantify mRNA, the ΔCt values (ΔCt = Ct target – Ct reference) obtained were normalized to the housekeeping β-actin gene *ACTB* for each of the target genes studied (*GNPTAB*, *GNPTG,* and *NAGPA*) and is shown in the plot (**Figure 17**). The data suggest that there is variability within the controls (father, mother, and sister) and there is no obvious difference between the proband and the internal control group.

The 2^- ΔΔCt calculations were performed to check if the control data can be pooled. The ΔΔCt value was obtained by subtracting the ΔCt of a proband with ΔCt of control (ΔΔCt = ΔCt test sample – ΔCt control). Because of the variability, and small sample size, 2^-ΔΔCt calculation, and statistical significance testing were not feasible. However, the data suggest that the expression of *GNPTG*, as well as *GNPTAB* and *NAGPA* genes in the proband, are within the range of the controls.

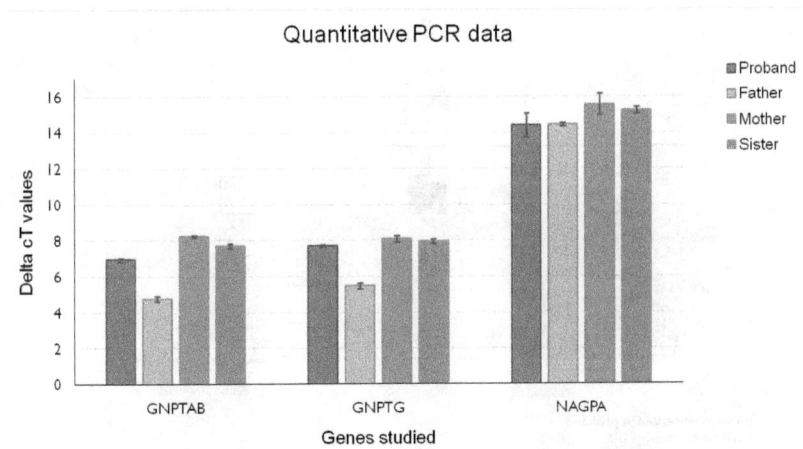

Figure 17: The relative levels of *GNPTG*, *GNPTAB*, and NAGPA mRNA expression were determined in WBC from blood sample of stuttering patients by real-time PCR normalized to β-actin expression. Data indicates ΔCt values ±SD

(iii) **Family STU 34**

The 15-year-old male proband with stuttering born to non consanguineous parents was ascertained from a National high school in Salem, Tamil Nadu, and had no complications during his birth. The age at onset of stuttering was unknown and reported as sudden and is right handed with good academic performance. Severity assessment rated him as severe with prolongations, blocks, irregular breathing and with difficulties in initial syllables. Secondary behaviours were mild. There was a situational increase in the stuttering such as in a classroom, while speaking with teachers, etc.

Mutation analysis identified a **heterozygous variant p. Arg44Pro in exon 2 of the *NAGPA* gene.** Extended testing and analysis revealed the presence of this variant in his unaffected father and his two unaffected brothers (Figure 18). Also, ACMG classifies this variant as benign.

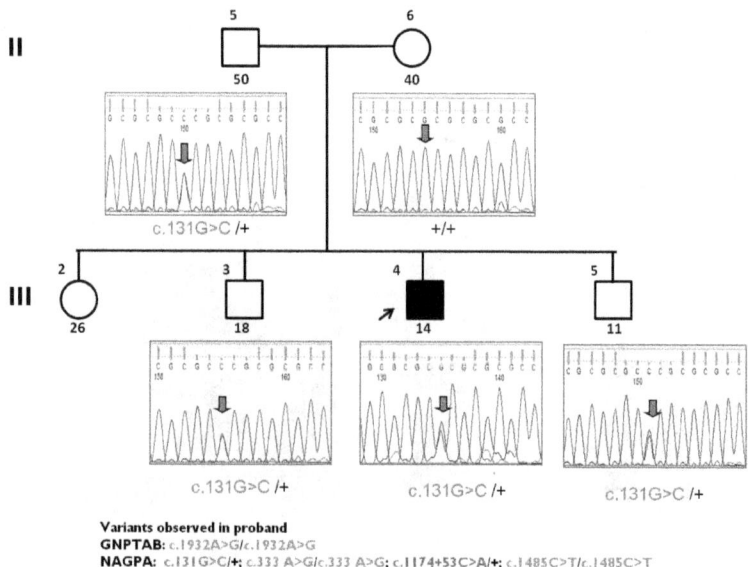

Figure 18: Partial chromatogram of c.131G>C (Arg44Pro) mutation in *NAGPA* gene

Table 22 lists a comprehensive variant profile observed in the three putative stuttering implicated genes in all the three probands presented above. The genes are known to be functionally related and belong to the lysosomal targeting pathway. On examining the variant profiles of these three probands (STU 29, STU 63, and STU 34) there was a co-occurrence of synonymous and non-coding variants with unknown clinical significance.

Chapter 4 *Results*

Table 22: Variant profile of the probands in the three putative genes for stuttering

SAMPLE	GNPTAB		GNPTG		NAGPA	
	HET	HOMO	HET	HOMO	HET	HOMO
STU 29	c.3598G>A (E19)	c.1932A>G (E 13)			c.333 A>G (E2)	c. 1485C>T (E10)
					c.1174+53C>A (I7)	
STU 63		c.1932A>G (E 13)	c.802A>C (E10)			c.333 A>G (E2)
						c. 1485C>T (E10)
						c.1174+53C>A (I 7)
STU 34		c.1932A>G (E 13)			c.131G>C(E2)	c.333 A>G (E2)
					c.1174+53C>A (I7)	c. 1485C>T (E10)

Bioinformatic analysis of the alignment of the secondary structure of mutated GNPTAB protein (p. Glu1200Lys) with the native protein identified loss of helix and addition of turn near the mutated region Figure 19a. A similar analysis for GNPTG protein (p. Ile268Leu) showed that the mutation did not affect the secondary structure (Figure 19b).

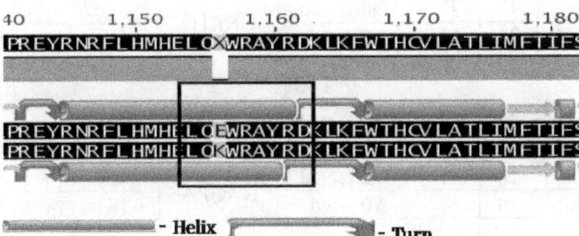

Figure 19a: MAFFT alignment of native and mutated secondary structure of GNPTAB protein using the Geneious Pro version 6.1.2 identified the loss of helix and addition of turn at the site of mutation.

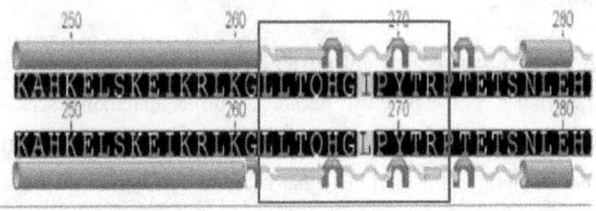

Figure 19b: MAFFT alignment of native and mutated secondary structure of GNPTG protein using the Geneious Pro version 6.1.2 showing no change in the secondary structure

Segregation analysis revealed that only one variant, p. Glu1200Lys in *GNPTAB* gene, co-segregated with the affected individual (**Table 23**) while p. Ile268Leu in *GNPTG* gene was found to be *de novo*. Since the *GNPTAB* variant is benign, the allele frequency of all likely causative variants was 0.8% (1/128) in the stuttering families studied.

Table 23: Segregation pattern and genotype-phenotype correlation of likely pathogenic variants identified in the three putative genes for stuttering among the 64 probands screened

Code	Individual	Age	Sex	Phenotype	Gene	Genotype	Remarks
STU 29							
II-2	Father	45	M	**Affected**		c.3598G>A/+	Cosegregation of the pathogenic allele suggests a dominant inheritance pattern
II-4	Mother	38	F	Unaffected		+/+	
III-4	Brother	20	M	**Affected**		c.3598G>A/+	
III-6	Sister	17	F	Unaffected	GNPTAB	+/+	
III-7	**Proband**	16	M	**Affected**		c.3598G>A/+	
III-8	Younger brother	15	M	Unaffected		+/+	Familial non consanguineous
STU 63							
II-5	Father	50	M	Unaffected		+/+	*de novo* variation
II-10	Mother	45	F	Unaffected	GNPTG	+/+	
III-1	**Proband**	24	M	**Affected**		c.802A>C/+	Sporadic non consanguineous
III-2	Sister	19	F	Unaffected		+/+	
STU 34							
II-5	Father	50	M	Unaffected		c.131G>C/+	The variation does not cosegregate with affected status
II-6	Mother	40	F	Unaffected		+/+	
III-3	Brother	18	M	Unaffected	NAGPA	c.131G>C/+	
III-4	**Proband**	14	M	**Affected**		c.131G>C/+	
III-5	Younger brother	11	M	Unaffected		DNA unavailable	Sporadic non consanguineous

■ indicates likely pathogenic missense variation

4.5.3 Exome sequencing

Stuttering being a complex disorder with strong heritability factor, emphasis was on molecular genetic studies, in the past two decades. Further mutational screening analysis of previously implicated genes (*GNPTAB*, *GNPTG* and *NAGPA*) that influence stuttering but ended up with a minimal resolution of 3.1% (2/64) that could be ascribed to these genes but remains inconclusive. The involvement of novel candidate genes in stuttering can certainly be addressed using next generation sequencing technology.

Exome sequencing (ES) in this study was performed in six individuals from two multiplex families with severe stuttering and the results of each family is presented in detail here. One family (STU 66) had affected subjects which is of affected parent-offspring category, while the second family (STU 65), constituted an affected sibling pair category.

Family STU 66

Family description

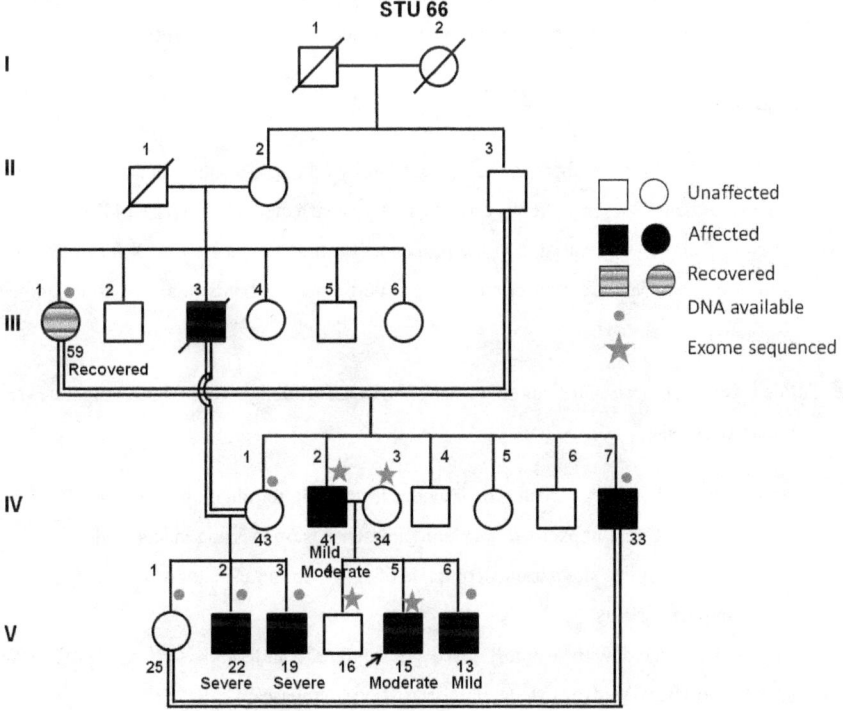

Figure 20: Five generation pedigree of stuttering family STU 66

From our existing school database of stuttering, a highly multiplex family was selected for ES studies in view of a plausible clue for heritability. This family was revisited in February 2018 and the pedigree was updated. This Telugu speaking family showed seven affected individuals across three generations with three inbreeding loops in the kindred (Figure 20). The proband (V-5) was born to non-consanguineous parents, where the father (IV-2) was affected with mild stuttering as observed during the time of investigation but the mother (IV-3) was unaffected. Both the proband (V-5) and his younger brother (V-6) had moderate stuttering with age at onset of 2.5 years that was progressive. The elder brother (V-4) of the proband was unaffected. In the extended family the grandfather, uncle (mild stuttering) and the first cousins of the proband were also affected with severe stuttering.

One nuclear family from these kindred was screened for exome sequencing comprising, affected father (IV-2), unaffected mother (IV-3), unaffected brother (V-4) and the proband (V-5).

Variant filtering

ES data of the four members in the nuclear family STU 66, resulted in a total of 73,426 variants in the affected father, 73,689 variants in the unaffected mother, 73,141 variants in unaffected sibling and 73,198 variants in the proband. Each of the individual variant files were subjected to defined variant filtering criteria, to profile the rare variants in all the four samples under investigation.

The defined filter comprises of three critical variants grouping *viz.*, high, moderate and intronic/direct splice site.

1. The high impact variant type includes frameshift, termination, start loss type,
2. The moderate impact variants being missense, stop loss and indels, and
3. Intronic splice site variants comprise of splice donor/acceptor or proximal splicing impact variants.

These variants are filtered with a cutoff for depth being 3X and MAF <1% in ExAC, 1000 genomes, and proprietary Medvar (Medgenome variation) databases.

Segregation analysis of variants

The variant prioritization and candidate gene identification in family-based cohort often rely on profiling the common and uncommon gene variants present in the affected and unaffected members in this family. An open source tool called InteractiVenn (Heberle et al., 2015) was deployed for this purpose that can handle up to six data sets (creates Venn diagram). A mean of 2245 variants (ranging from 2188-2296) were analyzed and all possible subsets of the data between the four sequenced individuals in the family produced a number of regions that were unique based on the combinations (Figure 21).

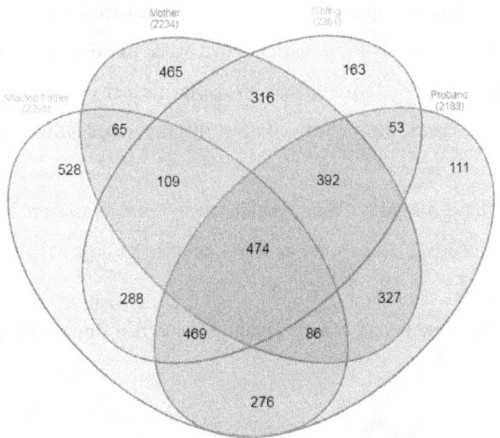

Figure 21: Venn diagram showing the variants shared among the four individuals in the STU 66 family (15 combinations)

It was observed that 276 genes were common to both affected father and the proband. The filtered variants in the 276 common genes were subjected to downstream analysis as depicted below in the flow chart (Figure 22). Given the common set of genes, the variant detected in each of these affected individuals may not be the same, but are absent in the unaffected mother and unaffected brother. Those variants were further sorted for its commonness in both affected father and the proband, ensuing in 260 such common variants harbored in 248 genes.

Irrespective of the variant types, further filtering was done based on known and novel variants. Of these 260 common variants, 217 were previously known (with identifiers in the literature or in dbSNP database with rsIDs) and 43 were novel variants (hitherto unreported in any of the previously described variant resource database). However, only 84 of the 217 known variants and 13 out of the 43 novel variants fall in the coding region. In our exhaustive analysis, no significant intronic/UTR variations were detected other than the missense variations and indels.

Exclusion criteria

The 84 known variants were filtered using the exclusion criteria described below:

(i) those **predicted as tolerant** using MetaSVM (meta-analytic support vector machine (SVM)) and MetaLR which accommodate multiple omics data to detect consensus genes associated with disease, were excluded. In other words those variants that were **predicted to be damaging** by atleast one or more than one prediction tool was considered for further validation.

(ii) In sorting the phenotype, variants in gene with completely unmatched OMIM phenotypes were excluded.

(iii) Proximal splice site variants placed at >8 nucleotides away from exon were also excluded.

(iv) Variants in zinc finger encoding genes were as well excluded as they have very omnipresent role.

Application of the above exclusion criteria resulted to **narrow down 18 variants from 84 known variants.**

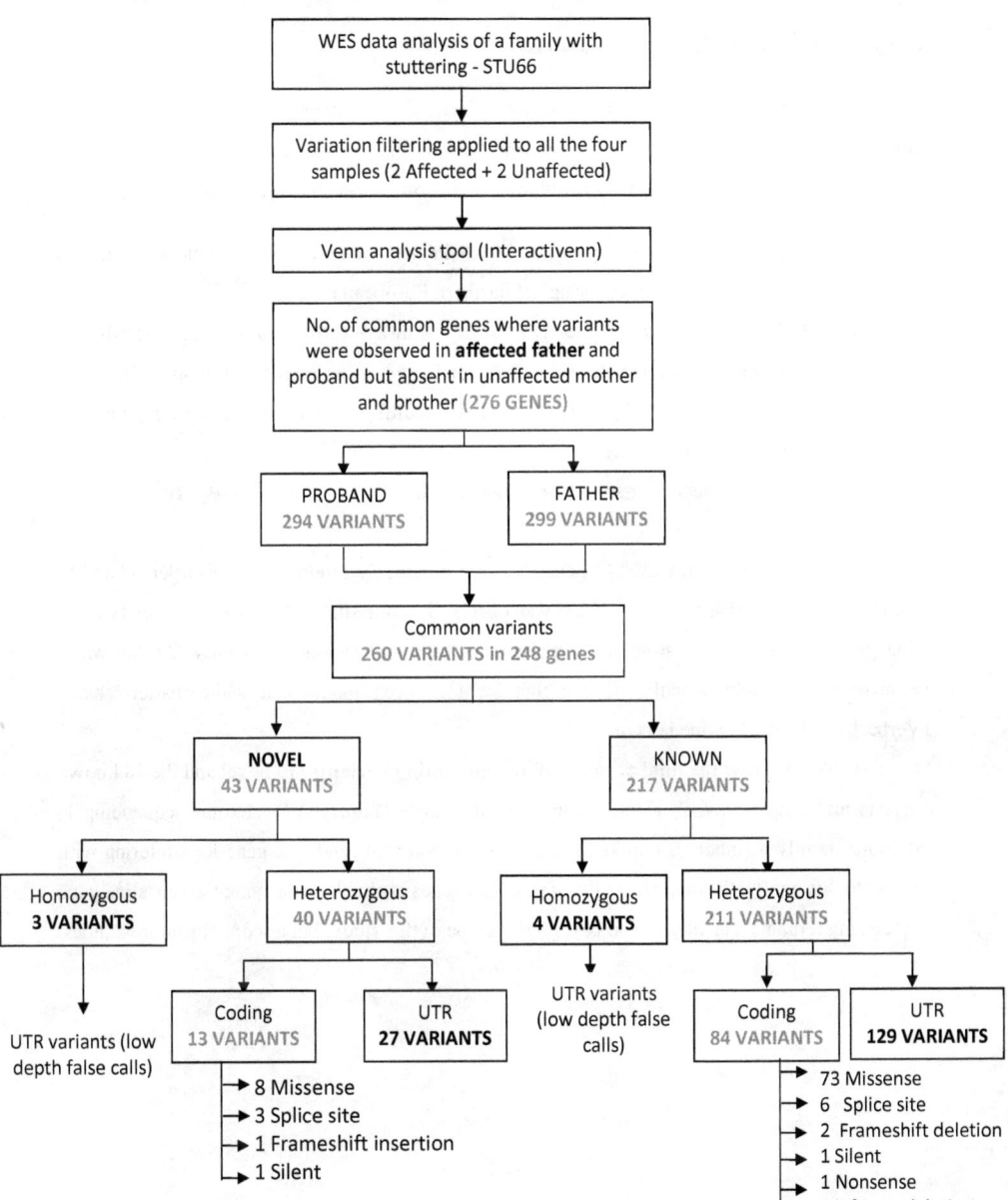

Figure 22: Bioinformatic-analysis pipeline applied to exome sequence data of a STU 66 family with stuttering

Variants compared with previous databases

These 18 shortlisted variants were taken forward for further scrutiny referring to three databases, in order to identify for the presence of variants in our study that match with the previously reported genes attributed to stuttering or any other speech and language disorders:

1. Significant SNPs reported by Kraft (2010) in the 'Genome-wide association study of persistent developmental stuttering' of northern European ancestry.
2. The 123 genes listed in the lysosomal pathway (https://pathcards.genecards.org/card/lysosome). Since the three genes so far known to be implicated in stuttering were identified in the lysosomal pathway, this study carefully observed any potential variants in genes related to this pathway.
3. The genes so far listed for speech and language disorders by Guerra *et.al.*, (2019)

Only one variant in *COL4A2* gene that was previously reported in a disorder related to fluency of language (Eicher *et al.*, 2013) was observed in our study. *COL4A2* encodes type IV collagen that forms a major structural component of basement membrane. *COL4A2* is known to be involved in cerebrovascular disease that include porencephaly and white matter lesions (Verbeek *et al.*, 2012; Yoneda *et al.*, 2012).

Table 24 shows the **final account of 31 segregating variants** (13 novel and the 18 known variants including *COL4A2*) identified **in STU 66 family (Figure A7).** Exome sequencing in additional family members is required to arrive at the potential candidate gene for stuttering with respect to this family. With the huge list of potential genes available identifying the causative gene segregating remains a challenge and beyond the scope of this study, but a scope for future studies.

Table 24: Compilation of the variants common in parent offspring pair of STU 66 family correlating to speech language disorders that includes 15 novel variants observed along with the bioinformatic predictions for pathogenicity

S.No	Variant	Zygosity	Gene	dbSNP ID/Novel	Var Class	AA Change	cDNA Change	Transcript	Depth (ALT%)	Meta SVM	MetaLR	SIFT	PP2 (HDiv/HVar)	ExAC (All)
					NOVEL CODING VARIANTS IDENTIFIED IN THE PRESENT STUDY									
1	chr1:15988026C>CAC	HET	RSC1A1	Novel	FRAMESHIFT-INS	p.Arg582ThrfsTer23	c.1665_1743dup	ENST00000345034.1/1	198 (36.1446%)	NA	NA	NA	NA/NA	NA
2	chr16:57702318G>T	HET	GPR97	Novel	INTRONIC-SS-DNR	NA	c.58+1G>T	ENST00000333493.4/1	31 (45.1613%)	NA	NA	NA	NA/NA	NA
3	chr8:192780011T>G	HET	CSGALNACT1	Novel	MISSENSE	p.Ile328Leu	c.982A>C	ENST00000454498.2/7	20 (45.0000%)	T	T	T	BN/NA	NA
4	chr19:45911978A>C	HET	CD3EAP	Novel	MISSENSE	p.Lys251Thr	c.752A>C	ENST00000309424.3/3	51 (50.0000%)	NA	NA	D	PrD/NA	NA
5	chr3:64619379C>T	HET	ADAMTS9	Novel	MISSENSE	p.Ser678Asn	c.2033G>A	ENST00000498707.1/13	144 (54.8611%)	T	T	D	BN/NA	NA
6	chr15:42156102C>A	HET	SPTBN5	Novel	INTRONIC-SS-DNR-PRX	NA	c.7034+5G>T	ENST00000209556.6/40	137 (43.7956%)	T	T	NA	NA/NA	NA
7	chr8:28956685G>A	HET	KIF13B	Novel	MISSENSE	p.Ser1430Phe	c.4289C>T	ENST00000241891.7/36	66 (62.1212%)	NA	NA	T	BN/NA	NA
8	chr8:144789722C>A	HET	CCDC166	Novel	MISSENSE	p.Gln154His	c.462G>T	ENST00000542437.1/2	61 (37.7049%)	NA	NA	T	PoD/NA	NA
9	chr3:126747829C>T	HET	PLXNA1	Novel	INTRONIC-SS-ACR-PRX	NA	c.4670-7C>T	ENST00000393409.2/24	157 (57.0513%)	T	T	NA	NA/NA	NA
10	chr15:52074948G>T	HET	TMOD2	Novel	MISSENSE	p.Ala219Ser	c.655G>T	ENST00000497004.7	87 (49.4253%)	T	T	T	PrD/NA	NA
11	chr16:50667104C>T	HET	NKD1	Novel	SILENT-SS-PRX	p.Gly275(=)	c.825C>T	ENST00000268459.9/10	111 (42.3423%)	NA	NA	NA	NA/NA	NA
12	chr1:118260011G>T	HET	C1orf167	Novel	MISSENSE	p.Gly243Val	c.728G>T	ENST00000433342.1/3	102 (52.0000%)	NA	NA	D	PrD/NA	NA
13	chr19:12089178C>G	HET	ZNF763	Novel	MISSENSE	p.Gln167Glu	c.499C>G	ENST00000590798.1/4	283 (52.1277%)	T	T	D	PoD/NA	NA
					KNOWN VARIANTS IDENTIFIED IN THE STUDY									
14	chr1:21952802G>T	HET	RAP1GAP	rs546205260	MISSENSE	p.Pro577Thr	c.169C>A	ENST00000290101.4/3	48 (37.5000%)	D	D	T	BN/NA	0.00050908
15	chr1:133160566A>G	HET	SYNC	rs545336096	MISSENSE	p.Leu378Pro	c.1133T>C	ENST00000409190.3/2	55 (47.2727%)	D	D	D	PrD/NA	0.00017302
16	chr2:238245052CACAGGCTTTGTTGTGGTGGT>C	HET	COL6A3	rs746284792	INFRAME-DEL	p.Thr2892_Thr2898del	c.8670_8690del	ENST00000295550.4/40	187 (43.5294%)	NA	NA	NA	NA/NA	0.00061783

Chapter 4 — Results

S.No	Variant	Zygosity	Gene	dbSNP ID	Var Class	AA Change	cDNA Change	Transcript	Depth (ALT%)	Meta SVM	MetaL R	SIFT	PP2 (HDiv/HVar)	ExAC (All)
17	chr3:52233273C>T	HET	ALAS1	rs757391785	MISSENSE	p.Arg6Cys	c.16C>T	ENST00000094965.2/3	127 (49.6063%)	D	D	D_lc	PrD/NA	0.0001237
18	chr5:1596964498G>A	HET	CCNJL	rs904712173	MISSENSE	p.Arg157Cys	c.469C>T	ENST00000005287.2/4	134 (47.7612%)	NA	NA	D_lc	BN/NA	5
19	chr7:48378053G>A	HET	ABCA13	rs569177123	INTRONIC-SS-DNR	NA	c.10204+1G>A	ENST00000358031/29	111 (44.1441%)	NA	NA	NA	NA/NA	0.00063778
20	chr7:148311155A>G	HET	C7orf33	rs546618103	MISSENSE	p.Met76Val	c.226A>G	ENST00000007003.2/2	30 (36.6667%)	NA	NA	T_lc	BN/NA	0.00053652
21	chr10:31710097G>A	HET	LOC101927848	rs139771837	MISSENSE	p.Pro132Ser	c.394C>T	XM_005252648.1/1	9 (66.6667%)	NA	NA	NA	NA/NA	NA
22	chr12:2112036778GC>G	HET	ATXN2	rs757862555	FRAMESHIFT-DEL	p.Gln180HisfsTer26	c.540del	ENST00000776173/1	18 (26.6667%)	NA	NA	NA	NA/NA	0.00719089
23	chr12:1120367807GTGCTGCTGC>T	HET	ATXN2	rs752859349	FRAMESHIFT-DEL	p.Gln177AlafsTer69	c.528_538del	ENST00000776173/1	21 (23.5294%)	NA	NA	NA	NA/NA	0.00211864
24	chr13:9904310A>G	HET	FARP1	rs547864277	MISSENSE	p.Glu353Gly	c.1058A>G	ENST00000195626/11	94 (47.8723%)	D	D	T	PrD/NA	0.00003296
25	chr13:11110809 14G>A	HET	COL4A2	rs375700657	MISSENSE	p.Gly154Glu	c.461G>A	ENST00000604675/7	49 (59.1837%)	D	D	D	PrD/NA	0.00016815
26	chr15:23014502C>T	HET	NIPA2	rs150146701	MISSENSE	p.Ala75Thr	c.223G>A	ENST00000374513/6	61 (57.3770%)	NA	NA	T	PoD/NA	0.00014797
27	chr15:40544858C>A	HET	C15orf56	rs568969059	INTRONIC-SS-DNR	NA	c.231+1G>T	ENST00000195033/1	101 (45.9184%)	NA	NA	NA	NA/NA	0.00131637
28	chr16:1458529T>C	HET	UNKL	rs556641262	MISSENSE	p.Tyr103Cys	c.308A>G	ENST00000974621/3	14 (50.0000%)	NA	NA	D_lc	BN/NA	0.00128205
29	chr16:2580768C>A	HET	CEMP1	rs535834483	MISSENSE	p.Ala103Ser	c.307G>T	ENST00000823501/1	166 (44.2424%)	NA	NA	D_lc	PoD/NA	0.00088222
30	chr19:17163775G>A	HET	HAUS8	rs373920841	SILENT-SS-PRX	p.Asp263(=)	c.789C>T	ENST00000536695/10	91 (43.9560%)	NA	NA	NA	NA/NA	0.00017304
31	chr19:40149104G>A	HET	LGALS16	rs774653270	MISSENSE	p.Glu31Lys	c.97G>A	ENST00000920513/3	89 (62.9213%)	NA	NA	T	BN/NA	0.000018

Family STU 65
Family description

From our existing school database of stuttering another highly multiplex family was taken up for ES to increase the chance of finding any genes specific to this ethnicity. This family was revisited in November 2017 and updated. This Tamil speaking family belongs to a predominant endogamous Mudaliar caste group. This family has more than 20 affected individuals spread across six generations as well. The extended family has many clusters each with several nuclear families showing subjects with stuttering status. The expansion and documentation of the familial history was possible due to the availability of a number of senior informants starting from the third generation. There is an intense multigenerational inbreeding tracing the stuttering phenotype back to a common female founder (Figure 23).

The proband (V-33) and his affected brother (V-35) were born to consanguineous parents (first cousins once removed) with another inbreeding loop in parents on maternal side of the proband. Both the parents were affected [father (III-21) and mother (IV-8)] with mild stuttering during the time of investigation. Though the mother had severe stuttering in her young age, now her dysfluencies have reduced but her speech rate was observed to be fast. Jaw clenching was observed at rest and during conversation. Father also had repetitions and jaw clenching.

Both the proband (V-33) and his younger brother (V-35) had developed stuttering gradually with age at onset of 2.5 years and were assessed to be moderate and severe. Mother did not report any complications during their birth and both of them were right-handed. The proband stopped his schooling by 10th standard and had situational increase of stuttering when speaking to strangers. Dysfluencies observed includes hard contacts in initial syllable, prolongation, silent pauses, syllable and part-word repetitions with iterations of 2-3. His secondary behaviours included eye blinks, clicking sounds, fixed articulatory posture, nose flaring, tension in the neck, jaw jerking and left side head nod that was frequent. His rate of speech was slow and intelligibility in speech was fair.

Proband sibling was also assessed to be severe with repetitions and prolongations along with secondary features like eye blinking, facial grimace, hand fidgeting, etc. He also had situational increase in stuttering at office, to his superiors, when excited or afraid but continued beyond school education.

Figure 23: Six generational pedigree of a stuttering family STU 66

In the extended family the grandmother (mild) and his maternal aunts were also affected. The cousins of the proband were also affected with severe stuttering. The family members in the kindred have been extensively phenotyped (Table 25).

Variant prioritization

On sequencing, the two affected individuals (V-33, proband) and (V-35, affected brother) in the family, a total of 58,346 and 51,062 exonic and splice site variants were detected respectively. The variants analysis files of the two affected individuals in this family were subjected to variant filtering to profile the rare variants common to both sibs under investigation. The filter sorts out high impact, moderate impact and splice variants as explained above, with a depth of 3X and MAF <1% in ExAC, 1000 genomes and Medvar (Medgenome variation) databases. In this way the filter analysis identified 365 variants in the affected brother.

Segregation of variants in affected members

The whole variant data of proband and the 365 variants obtained for the affected brother were subjected to InteractiVenn, that gives the unique and common genes between the sib-pair. It was observed that **294 genes were common** to both siblings wherein a variant that existed may or may not be the same variant (Figure 24). The downstream analysis of the variants observed in the 294 common genes (to start with) is depicted in the flow chart (Figure 25). The variants observed were further sorted out to identify those variants that were common to both sibs. We observed **161 such common variants** harbored on 153 genes. Of these 161 common variants, 156 were **known variants** and five were novel variants all of which were found in the coding regions.

A similar four step exclusion criteria were employed to scrutinize the 156 known variants that resulted in narrowing down of 29 variants, wherein four were homozygous and 25 were heterozygous variants (Figure A8). None of the 29 variants shortlisted in the present study were reported previously. However, in *NAGPA* gene variant that was already implicated in stuttering, a novel variant was identified.

Table 25: Characterization of the stuttering phenotype and other associated findings among 24 individuals examined in the STU 65 family

S.No	Code No	Relationship	Age (years)	Sex	Affected status	Dysfluencies	Secondary behaviours	Severity	Other findings	Remarks
1	65-1	Proband	35	M	Affected	Hard contacts in initial syllable, prolongation, silent pauses, syllable and part word repetitions, Iterations 2-3	Jaw jerks, head nods, clicking sounds, eyeblinks, fixed articulatory postures	Moderate	Avoidance and escape behaviours were observed. Rate of speech was slow	Speech intelligibility was fair with occasional repetitions required. No complication during delivery (normal)
2	65-2	Sibling	32	M	Affected	Repetitions and prolongations	Eye blinks, facial grimace, hand fidgeting	Severe	Anticipatory and escape behaviours were observed	Speech intelligibility was good
3	65-3	Father	68	M	Affected	Repetition	Lower jaw movement	Mild	Situational fear	-
4	IV-8 65-4	Mother	59	F	Affected	No significant dysfluencies were noticed.	Jaw clenching was observed at rest and during conversation	Mild	Rate of speech was fast. Breathing pattern was thoracic breathing and quick inhalation during speech	Speech intelligibility was fair and requires occasional repetitions to understand
5		Younger sibling	Deceased at 30 years	M	Mentally challenged	-	-	-	Epileptic seizures, MR, low set years, stunted growth, webbed neck, flat foot (Down syn?) speech and language impaired	Mother tried to abort using medicine.
6	IV-9 65-5	Uncle	65	M	Normal	-	-	-	-	-

S.No.	Code No	Relationship	Age (years)	Sex	Affected status	Dysfluencies	Secondary behaviours	Severity	Other findings	Remarks
7	IV-10 65-6	Maternal Aunt	58	F	Affected	Blocks, interjections	-	Very mild or recovered	Right hand thumb sucking for long period	Had severe stuttering until age 14 after which recovered gradually
8	V-12 65-7	Cousin	32	M	Affected	Hesitation, repetitions, blocks	Lower jaw movement tremor	Moderate	-	-
9	V-13 65-8	Cousin	29	F	Affected	Hesitation, repetitions, mild blocks	Eye blinking, gasping	Moderate	Situational fear	Faced teasing Has wheezing problem
10	IV-12 65-9	Uncle	60	M	Normal	-	-	-	-	-
11	IV-13 65-10	Maternal Aunt	56	F	Affected	Repetitions, Prolongations	Eye blinking	Mild	Difficulties in initial syllable Situational increase	Decreased after 23 years
12	V-13 65-11	Cousin	24	M	Affected	Repetitions, prolongation, interjections	Leg shaking, head nods	Mild	-	-
13	V-14 65-12	Cousin	21	F	Normal	-	-	-	-	-
14	III-1	Grand mother	deceased after phenotyping at 85years		Affected	Prolongations, syllable and part word repetitions with 2-3 iterations Occasional hard contacts No dysfluency during chants or prayers	Movement of legs and head nods, eyeblinks and jaw clenching were observed	Mild	Rate of speech was fast Had leprosy at the age of 5. All her children were born and fed when she had leprosy	Speech intelligibility was good
15	IV-6	Uncle	-	M	Normal	-	-	-	-	-

S.No.	Code No	Relationship	Age (years)	Sex	Affected status	Dysfluencies	Secondary behaviours	Severity	Other findings	Remarks
16	IV-7	Maternal aunt	-	F	Affected	Repetitions, blocks	-	Very mild	It was severe when she was young but now her dysfluency has decreased	Situational increase
17	V-9	Cousin	-	M	Affected	Repetitions	-	Mild	No birth complications. Studied till grade eight	Avoidance present
18	V-11	Cousin	-	M	Affected	Syllable repetition, silent pauses	-	Mild	No birth complications and no complications	Situational fear Avoidance present
19	IV-3	Uncle	deceased at 52 years	M	Normal	-	-	-	-	Deceased before the study
20	IV-4	Maternal aunt	-	F	Affected	Blocks and part word repetitions	-	Mild	Education till grade VIII. Was criticized in school	Reproductive history shows infant mortality. The third born girl baby died in 7 days after birth. Mother had malaria during the birth of this child
21	V-1	Cousin	-	M	Affected	Not able to meet him	-	-	No complications in delivery	-
21	V-3	Cousin	-	F	Normal	-	-	-	-	-
23	III-8	Grandmother	73	F	Affected	Repetitions, blocks	Lower jaw jerks	-	-	-
24	III-20	Maternal aunt	-	F	Mild hearing loss	No stuttering but reading disability	-	-	Speech delay. There was no speech until 9 years after which started to talk gibbrish and picked up speech gradually	Very sick infant history Had typhoid and jaundice at 1 1/2 years Skin problems

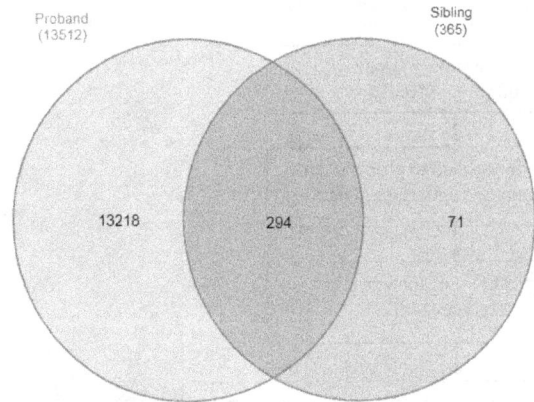

Figure 24: Venn diagram showing the variants shared between the affected sib pair in the STU 65 family

Table 26 shows the **final inventory of 34 variants** (29 known and five novel variants) identified **in STU 65 family**. However, exome sequencing in additional members and segregation analysis are required to discover the causative gene for stuttering with respect to this family.

Since the family had consanguinity for three generation it is worth to target the homozygous variants first. Hence looking closer at the homozygous variants only one homozygous *NLRP11* **gene variant** was present in both the sibs. Other homozygous variants status disagrees with sibs, that is if one sib is homozygous for a variant the other sib is heterozygous and vice versa. *NLRP11* **gene could be a possible candidate gene with respect to this family.** *NLRP11* is a member of NOD like receptor protein with N-terminal pyrin death domain (PYD), nucleoside triphosphate hydrolase domain (NACHT) and C-terminal leucine rich repeats (LRR). In general NLR proteins are responsible for inflammasome formation, though NLRP11 has pyrin domain responsible for formation of inflammasome it represses NF-κB and type I interferon responses, involved in inflammation pathways (Ellwanger *et al.,* 2018). Inflammation often is linked to dysfunction of immune system but neuro-immune and neuro- inflammation has been established as key factors in the development of Autism, where speech is also affected (Siniscalco et al., 2018).

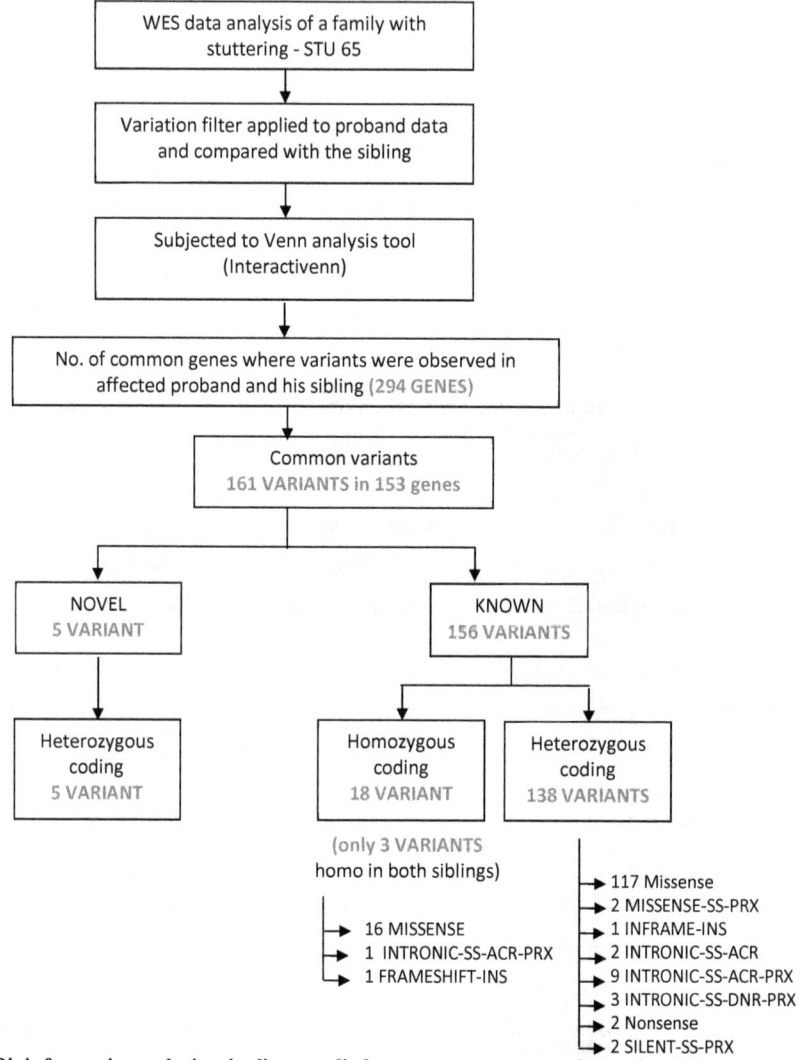

Figure 25: Bioinformatic-analysis pipeline applied to exome sequence data of a STU 65 family with stuttering

Table 26: Compilation of the variants common in sib pair of STU 65 family correlating to speech language disorders that includes 8 novel variants observed along with the bioinformatic predictions for pathogenicity

SNo	Variant	Zygosity	Gene	dbSNP ID	Var Class	AA Change	cDNA Change	Transcript	Depth (ALT%)	Meta SVM	MetaLR	SIFT	PP2 (HDiv/HVar)	ExAC (All)
\multicolumn{15}{l}{NOVEL CODING VARIANTS IDENTIFIED IN THE PRESENT STUDY (8 GENES)}
1	chr4:79229263G>T	HET	FRAS1	Novel	MISSENSE	p.Lys526Asn	c.1578G>T	ENST00000264895.6/15	127 (57.9365%)	T	T	T	BN/NA	NA
2	chr13:28851509 A>C	HET	PAN3	Novel	MISSENSE	p.Ile729Leu	c.2185A>C	ENST00000380958.3/15	165 (51.2500%)	T	T	T	PoD/NA	NA
3	chr16:5083494C>T	HET	NAGPA	Novel	MISSENSE	p.Glu108Lys	c.322G>A	ENST00000312251.3/2	59 (59.6491%)	T	NA	NA	PD/NA	NA
4	chr16:28842390 G>A	HET	ATXN2L	Novel	MISSENSE	p.Ala440Thr	c.1318G>A	ENST00000395547.2/10	57 (43.6364%)	T	T	T	BN/NA	NA
5	chr19:2991877C>G	HET	TLE6	Novel	MISSENSE	p.Ile427Met	c.1281C>G	ENST00000246112.4/14	96 (53.2609%)	NA	NA	T	BN/NA	NA
\multicolumn{15}{l}{KNOWN VARIANTS IDENTIFIED IN THE STUDY (29 GENES)}
6	chr2:231973941 T>A	HET	HTR2B	rs564438017	NONSENSE	p.Lys246Ter	c.736A>T	ENST00000258400.3/4	167 (57.2327%)	NA	NA	NA	NA/NA	0.000
7	chr3:49298212T>A	HET	RP11-3B7.1	rs537218816	MISSENSE	p.Val56Glu	c.167T>A	ENST00000440528.3/1	115 (42.8571%)	NA	NA	T	PoD/NA	0.000
8	chr6:170064371 G>A	HET	WDR27	rs551066667	MISSENSE	p.Ser180Leu	c.539C>T	ENST00000420344.2/6	63 (49.1525%)	NA	NA	D_lc	PoD/NA	0.000
9	chr7:31594088G>A	HET	CCDC129	rs768410299	INTRONIC-SS-ACR	NA	c.242-1G>A	ENST00000451887.2/2	130 (60.9375%)	NA	NA	NA	NA/NA	0.000
10	chr11:12273534 2A>C	HET	CRTAM	rs575784420	INTRONIC-SS-ACR	NA	c.734-2A>C	ENST00000227348.4/6	142 (56.3380%)	NA	NA	NA	NA/NA	0.000
11	chr13:33741684 G>T	HET	STARD13	rs765684140	INTRONIC-SS-DNR-PRX	NA	c.241+4C>A	ENST00000336934.5/2	135 (55.3846%)	NA	NA	NA	NA/NA	0.000
12	chr17:10417441 G>A	HET	MYH1	rs112621883	SILENT-SS-PRX	p.Thr178(=)	c.534C>T	ENST00000226207.5/7	250 (49.5833%)	NA	NA	NA	NA/NA	0.000
13	chr17:16331627 G>A	HET	TRPV2	rs201142576	INTRONIC-SS-ACR-PRX	NA	c.1351-4G>A	ENST00000338560.7/8	53 (52.8302%)	NA	NA	NA	NA/NA	0.003
14	chr20:60887690 C>T	HET	LAMA5	rs201429053	SILENT-SS-PRX	p.Pro3075(=)	c.9225G>A	ENST00000252999.3/67	174 (50.0000%)	NA	NA	NA	NA/NA	0.000
15	chrX:2833605C>T	HET	ARSD	rs111939179	NONSENSE	p.Trp331Ter	c.992G>A	ENST00000381154.1/6	34 (40.6250%)	NA	NA	NA	NA/NA	0.000
16	chr10:12819289 5G>GCGA	HET	C10orf90	rs577118647	INFRAME-INS	p.Ser291dup	c.871_873dup	ENST00000284694.7/3	206 (48.1675%)	NA	NA	NA	NA/NA	0.002

S.No	Variant	Zygosity	Gene	dbSNP ID	Var Class	AA Change	cDNA Change	Transcript	Depth (ALT%)	Meta SVM	MetaLR	SIFT	PP2 (HDiv/HVar)	ExAC (All)
17	chr17:4348389C>T	HET	SPNS3	rs146383415	MISSENSE	p.Arg110Cys	c.328C>T	ENST00000355530 2/3	135 (51.8797%)	D	D	D	PrD/NA	0.002
18	chr1:228645367 T>C	HET	HIST3H2A	rs533207092	MISSENSE	p.Tyr51Cys	c.152A>G	ENST00000366695 2/1	239 (50.8475%)	D	D	D_lc	PrD/NA	0.000
19	chr3:130380675 C>T	HET	COL6A6	rs374436074	MISSENSE	p.Arg2009Trp	c.6025C>T	ENST00000358511 6/34	114 (57.1429%)	NA	NA	D	PrD/NA	0.001
20	chr3:52800237T >C	HET	NEK4	rs143584767 1	MISSENSE	p.Tyr172Cys	c.515A>G	ENST00000233027 5/3	100 (59.1837%)	D	NA	D	PrD/NA	NA
21	chr8:104943573 G>A	HET	RIMS2	rs768216298	MISSENSE	p.Gly776Glu	c.2327G>A	ENST00000406091 3/12	29 (27.5862%)	NA	NA	D_lc	PrD/NA	0.000
22	chr12:417038C>A	HET	KDM5A	rs560791888	MISSENSE	p.Ser1171Ile	c.3512G>T	ENST00000399788 2/23	218 (37.6744%)	D	D	T	BN/NA	0.000
23	chr12:45059369 G>A	HOMO	NELL2	rs183846411	MISSENSE	p.Arg498Cys	c.1492C>T	ENST00000437801 2/14	211 (100.0000%)	D	D	T	PoD/NA	0.000
24	chr12:53012089 C>T	HOMO	KRT73	rs746640286	MISSENSE	p.Gly74Ser	c.220G>A	ENST00000305748 3/1	287 (100.0000%)	NA	NA	T	BN/NA	0.000
25	chr16:31367996 G>A	HET	ITGAX	rs373555641	MISSENSE	p.Gly65Asp	c.194G>A	ENST00000268296 4/3	73 (57.1429%)	D	D	T	PoD/NA	0.002
26	chr17:74276788 T>C	HET	QRICH2	rs561759535	MISSENSE	p.Lys1304Glu	c.3910A>G	ENST00000262765 5/10	102 (45.5446%)	NA	NA	T	PrD/NA	0.008
27	chr11:11739196 7C>T	HET	DSCAML1	rs745820564	MISSENSE	p.Arg424His	c.1271G>A	ENST00000321322 6/6	225 (50.6849%)	NA	NA	T	PrD/NA	0.000
28	chr19:56320924 C>T	HOMO	NLRP11	rs140988779	MISSENSE	p.Arg351Gln	c.1052G>A	ENST00000443188 1/5	93 (100.0000%)	NA	NA	T	BN/NA	0.001
29	chr15:42573272 G>A	HET	GANC	rs571874657	MISSENSE	p.Ser120Asn	c.359G>A	ENST00000440615 2/4	80 (48.7179%)	NA	NA	D	BN/NA	0.003
30	chr13:28552258 G>T	HET	URAD	rs566926473	MISSENSE	p.Asp169Glu	c.507C>A	ENST00000332715 5/2	45 (62.2222%)	NA	NA	T	BN/NA	0.004
31	chr8:81762036> T	HET	SGK223	rs372452888	MISSENSE	p.Gln1228Lys	c.3682C>A	ENST00000520004 1/6	186 (42.0455%)	NA	NA	T	PoD/NA	0.000
32	chr17:17062065 C>G	HOM	MPRIP	rs138508481	MISSENSE	p.Leu599Val	c.1795C>G	ENST00000395811 5/14	45 (100.0000%)	NA	NA	T	BN/NA	0.002
33	chr12:92382910 A>T	HET	C12orf79	rs76906203	MISSENSE	p.Phe32Ile	c.94T>A	ENST00000549802 1/3	168 (49.0909%)	NA	NA	D_lc	PoD/NA	0.005
34	chr12:97414066> T	HET	WNK1	rs562247853	MISSENSE	p.Pro757Leu	c.2270C>T	ENST00000530271 2/9	170 (45.7831%)	NA	NA	NA	BN/NA	0.001

Identification of possible candidate genes

Both the multiplex stuttering families had vast number of potential candidate genes. In an attempt to find the causative genes and the pathways involved in stuttering, bioinformatics approach was employed. The 64 genes identified in STU 66 (30 genes) and STU 65 (34 genes) families were subjected to two kinds of analysis

1. Exclusion of variants shown to be common in GnomAD database to narrow down the candidate genes
2. Identify high value target genes by looking for **common biological mechanisms** using integrative systems biology approaches

1. Exclusion of variants shown to be common in GnomAD database to narrow down the list of candidate genes

Considering stuttering to be a less common trait, a variant threshold with an allele count of more than 20 were excluded. In other words, we do not expect the heterozygous allele count or the heterozygyous variant carriers (>=20) to have the specific clinical phenotype (stuttering) in the GnomAD database. Applying this, the 64 genes in the list could be reduced to **35 genes**: 17 genes in STU 66 family and 18 genes in STU 65 family.

2. Identify high value target by looking for common biological mechanisms using integrative systems biology approaches

Stuttering is genetically heterogeneous and identifying high value target genes is complicated. One possibility to resolve this problem, is to look for **common biological mechanisms** using integrative systems biology approach. Hence the 65 variants spread across **64 genes** filtered in both families, were further analyzed using Reactome (https://reactome.org) which is a open source database of biological pathways. Further, the expression profile of the proteins encoded by these 64 genes were retrieved from Human Protein Atlas (http://www.proteinatlas.org) that show the distribution of the protein across major tissues or organs (Table A8 and A9).

The phenotypic relevance of the **64 genes** were manually checked to identify those genes that were involved in any given pathway. This resulted in nine putative pathways encompassing **41 genes** (out of 64 genes), that can be directly or indirectly linked to stuttering in the two families studied (Table 27). Intriguingly, the list of genes that are possible candidate genes for stuttering among the two families are different, but fitting into common pathways.

Table 27: Manually curated list of candidate* genes identified in 9 putative pathways, that can be directly or indirectly linked to stuttering, in the two families studied

S.No	Gene list from family STU 66	Pathways	Gene list from family STU 65
1	***SPTBN5**, PLXNA1, RAPIGAP*	neural developmental pathways	***COL6A6**, NELL2, DSCAML1*
2	***ADAMTS9**, **COL6A3**, COL4A2*	extra cellular matrix organisation/degradation	***LAMA5**, **COL6A6**, **ITGAX***
3	*TMOD2, SYNC*	muscle contraction	*MYH1*
4	*CD3EAP*	gene expression	-
5	***SPTBN5**, ZNF763, CCNJL, KIF13B, ATXN2*	signal transduction/ vesicle transport	*ATXN2L, HTR2B, STARD13, **MYH1**, **LAMA5**, NEK4, MRIP, KDM5A*
6	*RSC1A1, NIPA2*	transport of small molecules	*TRPV2, WNK1*
7	*CSGALNACT1, **ADAMTS9**, **SPTBN5**, ALAS1*	metabolism	*PAN3, ARSD, WDR27, HSIT3H2A*
8	*GPR97, **SPTBN5**, ABCA13, UNKL*	immune system	*CRTAM, **ITGAX**, NLRP11*
9	-	Lysosome enzyme targeting	*NAGPA*

Note: *The candidate genes proposed are exclusive to affected segregating in heterozygous status, except for *NLRP11* that segregates in the homozygous state; **bold** indicates genes involved in multiple pathways

Similarly, **enrichment pathway analysis** (a tool in reactome database that uses a statistical test (hypergeometric distribution) was carried out involving all the **64 deleterious and novel variants** identified in the two families. This determines whether certain pathways are over-represented (enriched) in the submitted data, not because of chance. It provides a probability score corrected for false discovery rate, using the Benjamani-Hochberg method (https://reactome.org). Interestingly, 25 most relevant pathways encompassing 14 genes, were sorted based on their p-value (Table 28). The distribution of 14 genes that are identified by the enrichment pathway analysis in the two families are shown in Table 29.

Thus, genes sorted out utilizing manually curated and enrichment pathway analysis were selected based on their recurrence in two independent pathway analyses. Hence on comparing the

Tables 27 and 29 it was feasible to enrich the gene list from 41 to **14 genes** and most of the remaining genes are indicated as interactors.

The genes that interact significantly tend to have a common function and may be involved in the same pathway. Hence functional discussion of the 14 possible candidate genes were detailed to identify the pathways related to stuttering. The genes like *COL4A2, COL6A3, COL6A6* are involved in **formation and degradation of collagens** (Haq *et al.*, 2019), *ITGAX* for **integrin** (Takada *et al.*, 2007) and *LAMA5* for **laminin** (Maselli *et al.*, 2018). All of this form the extra cellular matrix (ECM) components. *ADAMTS9* gene codes for metalloproteinase involved in **ECM degradation** (Kelwick *et al.*, 2015). *CSGALNACT1* is involved in chondroitin sulfate biosynthesis, one of the GAGs associated to core protein as proteoglycans that also form the **component of ECM** (Uyama *et al.*, 2003).

Other genes observed in the present study were *TMOD2* involved in muscle contraction, *HTR2B* in signaling involving serotonin receptors, *RSC1A1, TRPV2 and WNK1* genes are engaged in transport of small molecules in stimuli-sensing channels. All the above genes might be involved in communication between neuron, muscle cells at NMJ and may coordinate production of speech.

ARSD belongs to cluster of sulfatase genes that hydrolyse GAGs and differs from other sulfatase genes and was found to represent truncated pseudogenes (Meroni *et al.*, 1996). *SPTBN5* is involved in vesicle transport and NCAM (neural cell adhesion molecule) signaling that plays important role in nervous system development and synaptic plasticity (Kleene *et al.*, 2010). Already implicated *NAGPA* genes identified in the study is involved in transport of lysosomal enzymes to lysososmes.

On dissecting the functional discussion of these 14 genes, an interesting link with **extra cellular matrix components and its function** was identified.

Table 28: Over-representation analysis results of variants identified in two ES families showing 25 most significant pathways related to stuttering using Reactome database

Pathway name	Entities				Reactions	
	found	ratio	p-value	FDR*	found	ratio
ECM proteoglycans	5 / 118	0.006	1.24e-04	0.047	5 / 23	0.002
Collagen chain trimerization	3 / 44	0.002	7.90e-04	0.149	2 / 28	0.002
Degradation of the extracellular matrix	5 / 210	0.01	0.002	0.172	6 / 105	0.009
The activation of arylsulfatases	2 / 17	8.36e-04	0.002	0.172	1 / 2	1.62e-04
NCAM1 interactions	3 / 64	0.003	0.002	0.172	1 / 10	8.12e-04
Collagen degradation	3 / 76	0.004	0.004	0.223	4 / 34	0.003
Assembly of collagen fibrils and other multimeric structures	3 / 79	0.004	0.004	0.223	3 / 26	0.002
Laminin interactions	2 / 33	0.002	0.008	0.377	11 / 15	0.001
Collagen biosynthesis and modifying enzymes	3 / 110	0.005	0.01	0.429	22 / 51	0.004
NCAM signaling for neurite outgrowth	4 / 223	0.011	0.013	0.451	8 / 23	0.002
Striated Muscle Contraction	2 / 43	0.002	0.013	0.451	4 / 4	3.25e-04
Collagen formation	3 / 150	0.007	0.023	0.656	25 / 77	0.006
Interleukin-4 and Interleukin-13 signaling	4 / 339	0.017	0.049	0.656	2 / 46	0.004
Gamma carboxylation, hypusine formation and arylsulfatase activation	2 / 89	0.004	0.051	0.656	1 / 39	0.003
Serotonin receptors	1 / 13	6.39e-04	0.051	0.656	1 / 3	2.44e-04
Anchoring fibril formation	1 / 15	7.38e-04	0.059	0.656	1 / 4	3.25e-04
Integrin cell surface interactions	4 / 362	0.018	0.059	0.656	7 / 54	0.004
Intestinal hexose absorption	1 / 22	0.001	0.085	0.656	1 / 3	2.44e-04
Glycosphingolipid metabolism	3 / 124	0.006	0.09	0.656	2 / 32	0.003
Crosslinking of collagen fibrils	1 / 24	0.001	0.092	0.656	1 / 13	0.001
Chondroitin sulfate biosynthesis	1 / 27	0.001	0.103	0.656	1 / 9	7.31e-04
Stimuli-sensing channels	2 / 136	0.007	0.105	0.656	2 / 25	0.002
Intestinal absorption	1 / 28	0.001	0.107	0.656	1 / 6	4.87e-04
Extracellular matrix organization	6 / 842	0.041	0.125	0.656	58 / 318	0.026
TRP channels	1 / 33	0.002	0.125	0.656	1 / 2	1.62e-04

* False Discovery Rate

Table 29: Tentative list of candidate* genes identified in enrichment pathways, that can be directly or indirectly linked to stuttering, in the two families studied

S.No	Gene list from family STU 66	Pathways	Gene list from family STU 65
1	COL4A2, COL6A3	ECM proteoglycans	COL6A6, ITGAX, LAMA5
2	COL4A2, COL6A3,	Collagen chain trimerization	COL6A6
3	ADAMTS9, COL4A2, COL6A3,	Degradation of the extracellular matrix	COL6A6, LAMA5
4	COL4A2, COL6A3,	The activation of arylsulfatases	COL6A6
5	COL4A2, COL6A3	Collagen degradation	COL6A6
6	COL4A2, COL6A3,	Assembly of collagen fibrils and other multimeric structures	COL6A6,
7	COL4A2	Laminin interactions	LAMA5
8	COL4A2, COL6A3,	Collagen biosynthesis and modifying enzymes	COL6A6
10	COL4A2, COL6A3, SPTBN5	NCAM signaling for neurite out-growth	COL6A6
11	TMOD2	Striated Muscle Contraction	
12	COL4A2, COL6A3,	Collagen formation	COL6A6,
13		Interleukin-4 and Interleukin-13 signaling	ITGAX, LAMA5
14		Gamma carboxylation, hypusine formation and arylsulfatase activation	ARSD
15		Serotonin receptors	HTR2B
16	COL4A2	Anchoring fibril formation	
17	COL4A2, COL6A3	Integrin cell surface interactions	COL6A6, ITGAX
18	RSC1A1	Intestinal hexose absorption	
19	ARSD	Glycosphingolipid metabolism	
20	COL4A2	Crosslinking of collagen fibrils	
21	CSGALNACT1	Chondroitin sulfate biosynthesis	
22		Stimuli-sensing channels	TRPV2, WNK1
23	RSC1A1	Intestinal absorption	
24	COL4A2, COL6A3	Extracellular matrix organization	COL6A6, ITGAX, LAMA5
25		TRP channels	TRPV2

Note: *The candidate genes proposed are exclusive to affected segregating in heterozygous status

Genes commonly observed among two multiplex stuttering families

To understand the genes that could cause stuttering the expansive list of genes with variations, that was exclusive to the affected individuals in each family was compared (276 genes in STU 66 family and 294 in STU 65). Irrespective of the variants, only seven genes were found to be common to both families (Figure 26). They are *SLC36A1, C1orf167, SYNC, TM4SF1, MUC6, SPTBN5* and *MSRB1*. Multiple variants were observed for each gene in all the affected members.

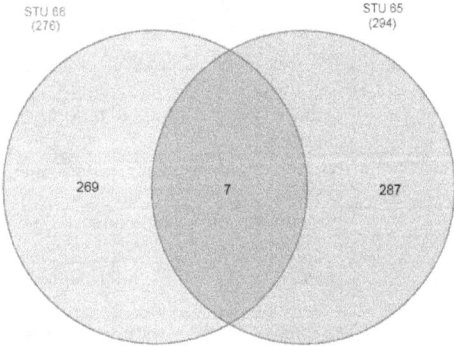

Figure 26: Venn diagram showing the genes shared between two stuttering multiplex families

On exploring the functions of these genes, it was found that *SLC36A1* gene encodes a proton dependent amino acid transporter which is highly expressed in brain. Mutation in this gene is associated with iminoglycinuria and spinocerebellar ataxia 45 that also involves poor coordination of **speech**. *C1orf167* encodes an uncharacterized protein associated with neural tube defects. *SYNC* gene that is highly expressed in muscle is involved in **muscle contraction** and is regarded as a marker of neuromuscular disease. *TM4SF1* and *MUC6* form the **extracellular component**. *SPTBN5* encodes protein that links membrane lipids, proteins and cytosolic factors to **cytoskeletal filaments** and also binds to kinesin and actin proteins. *MSRB1* gene acts in response to **stress** and is also involved in actin repolymerization.

Though all the above genes do not directly link with each other they seem to be involved in within cell or cell-cell communication at neuromuscular junction.

CHAPTER 5

DISCUSSION

5.1 GENETIC EPIDEMIOLOGY

Every country needs a credible estimate for the prevalence of stuttering to frame its national policy and effectively tackle the disorder in terms of management. Our study is the first targeted approach to scrutinize the prevalence of stuttering in India. The strengths of the study include broad and inclusive subject ascertainment, a relatively large sample size, and professional speech evaluation with high quality phenotype information. Stuttering was confirmed by investigators/speech pathologists, reconfirmed by parents, teachers and by self-report where available. Yet those who went undetected, e.g. with mild CWS, may create underestimate of the overall prevalence.

5.1.1 School data

It has been reported that the prevalence of stuttering ranged from 0.3% to 15.4% across different studies (Felsenfeld *et al.*, 2000), and the **prevalence** estimate in our study **(0.46%)** is substantially lower than the approximate mean prevalence of 1% (Bloodstein & Ratner, 2008). If the prevalence is indeed less than 1%, natural recovery may have ameliorated a greater initial risk of exhibiting stuttering (Yairi & Ambrose, 2013). Interestingly, a study that covered the life span from 1-99 years yielded an overall prevalence of 0.72%, with variation observed for discrete age groups (Craig *et al.*, 2002).

Gender is one of the strongest predisposing factors. Kidd (1984) suggests that the gender effect requires a lower threshold for males with females requiring more genetic loading and/or environmental forces for expression of the disorder. The increase in the male to female ratio with age is critical in understanding persistence and recovery (Ambrose *et al.*, 1997). We found that **recovery** reported among female affected relatives of the probands in general was high, and also observed that the classical male-favored sex ratio increased with age up to 9:1. The sex ratio of affected relatives is 4:1 in the families of male probands but decreases to 2:1 in the families of female probands. Although mild stuttering is difficult to recognize (Mellon *et al.,* 1993), we observed a greater proportion of mild than moderate and severe types of the disorder. Examining the sex ratios in familial and sporadic probands, Drayna *et al.,* (1999) observed that in familial cases the sex ratio is approximately equal (1.5:1), but in sporadic families the male to female ratio was much higher (7:1). By comparison, we observed an unchanged sex ratio in both familial and sporadic (6:1) cases.

Reports on **onset** are variable, with estimates suggesting that the highest risk is observed under 3-8 years (Andrews, 1964; Onslow, 1992; Yairi & Ambrose, 1999). Our observations concur with study of Yairi (1999), having two peaks at 3 and 5 years with the maximum at 3 years. In the present study 7.8% were CWS with age at onset greater than 10 years. This may be due to interiorized stuttering, i.e. subjects who avoid speech and are unaware of their stuttering, which is difficult to distinguish from acquired stuttering (Michael & Clifford, 1983).

Yairi and Ambrose who observed children close to the onset pointed out that, gradual onset was associated with family history and sudden onset (44%) with severity of stuttering (Yairi & Ambrose, 1992). There is a strong trend towards sudden onset in recent studies that reported 40% (Yairi & Ambrose, 2005), 50% (Reilly *et al.,* 2009) to 53% (Buck *et al.,* 2002). However, we observed only 27.2% CWS with gradual onset. In our study, while gradual onset was common in familial cases, sudden onset occurred in both familial and sporadic cases. However, our results may be confounded by inaccurate recall of parents in reporting age/manner of onset.

Familial incidence of stuttering (11%) is higher than the general population incidence (1%) supporting the genetic nature of stuttering. Male and female CWS had equal frequencies of affected relatives, with first degree relatives quite common, and in many previous studies a positive family history of 20-74% has been reported (Bloodstein, 1995). Kidd *et al.,* (1981) found that the relatives of female probands were affected more frequently than the relatives of male probands, but in our study male and female CWS had equal frequencies of affected relatives, in concordance with report by Ambrose *et al.,* (1993). Sporadic cases challenge the distinction between genetic and non-genetic that can ultimately be resolved by further studies.

Chapter 5 *Discussion*

Our population is characterized by substantial consanguinity, which can influence the expression of genetic disorders. However, it is important to emphasize that in assessing the impact of consanguinity on any disorder, a clear causal relationship needs to be established rather than reliance on speculation driven solely by the presence of close kin relationships in family pedigrees.

Although three large studies have reported on stuttering in school children worldwide (Boyle *et al.*, 2011), the possible role of parental **consanguinity** in stuttering has not previously been examined. We comprehensively evaluated parental consanguinity with an overall estimate of the mean inbreeding coefficient ($\alpha = 0.0165$), and observed a consanguinity rate of 22.6% among the parents of CWS, which closely approximates to that of general population of Tamil Nadu (22.4%) (Ramesh *et al.*, 1989). To better understand the influence of parental consanguinity, we compared our data with local and national level information on consanguineous marriage in India. All these reports are on the general population, i.e. without any known morbidity, and in South India consanguinity ranged from 7.5% in Kerala (Bittles *et al.*, 2002) to 54.9% in Pondicherry (Puri *et al.*, 1978) and up to 50% in rural Tamil Nadu (Rao *et al.*, 1972).

The **coefficient of inbreeding** (α) was highest among Hindus, because of the high rates of first cousin (33%) and uncle-niece marriages (33%). Although normal speaking parents predominated in our stuttering cohort, reflecting genetic heterogeneity, probands with at least one parent affected were not uncommon.

Stuttering probands included more first-born children, providing further evidence that stuttering is not a learned behavior (Wingate, 1971). Gladstien *et al.*, (1981) also reported previously that **birth order and age of separation** were not significant factors in the frequency of stuttering. The question of *caste* is potentially very interesting, but because of the large number of Hindu castes represented (n=36) and the low prevalence of stuttering no conclusions can be drawn.

Stuttering has been found to seriously affect personal relationships, limit career choices and lessen the individual's quality of life. Understanding **attitudinal differences** like behavioral reactions and the interaction with parents would help in counseling and the management of risk factors. In our population an awareness of speech therapy was poor, therefore there is a need to disseminate such information among probands/parents. Without appropriate education, parents tend to blame the child for being dysfluent on purpose. Hence counseling was directed to both the parent and child. We found CWS were withdrawn in speech activities. Interestingly, a majority of parents attributed prenatal elements as major contributors to stuttering. A previous study (Yairi *et al.,* 1996) on environmental influence was inconclusive.

On assessing the risk factors associated with severity, sex was significantly associated with severity, with female probands more likely to have a mild form of the disorder. A moderate effect was observed for increased severity with older age of onset. Family history and consanguinity within the pedigrees of probands were not associated with the severity of stuttering. This supports the findings of Yairi & Ambrose, (1999) that stuttering tends to cluster in families whereas severity does not. Thus, although there is an underlying genetic basis for stuttering, environmental factors also influence severity.

The **clustering of stuttering individuals** was present in the analyzed pedigrees, especially within consanguineous families. As expected, the kinship group test identified large proportions of closely related affected individuals in consanguineous families. The sibling recurrence risk is high for consanguineous families and differs significantly from non-consanguineous counterparts. These tests provide evidence of the **genetic nature** of the disorder, indicating that a rare gene variant may be responsible for its expression. The sibling recurrence risk is minimal though stuttering is quite prevalent in the population. It would be easier to identify a gene for larger risk ratio (Burmeister, 1999); but stuttering in contrary may have complex interaction of several genes, influence of environmental factors, gene-environment interactions and also epigenetic factors that cannot be ignored. The impact of consanguinity may have a very small effect in the disorder if it is due to high levels of homozygosity in minor alleles contributing the phenotype.

5.1.2 Hospital data

Comparing the school and hospital data a similar trend was observed among sex ratio, age at onset, birth order and sibship size. Familial incidence is described as the proportion of affected relatives in a collection of all the relatives documented in 101 pedigrees with positive family history. In this manner 178 out of 1596 relatives ascertained were affected resulting in 9% familial incidence in school data which is slightly lower than that of school data (11%). Familial aggregation of affected relatives was also lower in hospital data. The difference observed in the familial aggregation in our two cohorts may be due to the difference in the ascertainment adopted. In the former it is a simple proband sampling from the general school population and in the latter, it is physician referral from a speech therapy clinic.

Both familial incidence and familial aggregation points to its heritable or environmental etiology or even infectious agents. Given the cost and complexity of identifying the disease-causing genes, this preliminary step is useful as it narrows the focus for upcoming genetic research (Baglietto *et al.*, 2006; Matthews *et al.*, 2008).

5.2.2 Mutational analysis of implicated genes in stuttering

The present study will be the first research report on the Indian stuttering cohort to be investigated on the recurrence and implication of three functionally related lysosomal enzyme targeting pathway genes, *GNPTAB*, *GNPTG*, and *NAGPA*. The present study will be the first research report on the Indian stuttering cohort to be investigated on the recurrence and implication of three functionally related lysosomal enzyme targeting pathway genes, *GNPTAB*, *GNPTG*, and *NAGPA*.

A meta-analysis from worldwide reports on unrelated PWS has identified 81 rare nonsynonymous coding variants, in either of the three putative genes, yielding a frequency of 16% (164/1013)(Raza et al., 2016). While we have observed four nonsynonymous coding variants that accounted for 6% (4/64) in the present study. Among the twelve variants identified, five of them (p. Glu1200Lys and p. Thr644Thr in *GNPTAB* and p. Arg44pro, p. Gly111Gly and p. Asn495Asn in *NAGPA*) were previously reported in stuttering population. One variant (p. Pro234Pro in *GNPTG*) was reported in mucolipidosis III. However, the remaining six variants (p. Ile268Leu, p. Thr271Thr, c.-4 C>T in *GNPTG* and p. Leu47Phe, p. Thr465Ile, c.1174+53C>A in *NAGPA*) were observed in the gnomAD public database. Three of the conserved nonsynonymous variants (p. Glu1200Lys in *GNPTAB*, p. Ile268leu in *GNPTG*, and p. Arg44Pro in *NAGPA* gene) that were considered for segregation analysis are discussed individually.

STU 29 family with c.3598G>A variant in *GNPTAB* gene

The fact that the highest linkage scores were obtained for the variant c.3598G>A in *GNPTAB* combined with the lack of another plausible genetic variant within the linkage interval highlighted that this may have had an increased risk of stuttering when this variant is present in either one or two copies (Kang et al., 2010). Fedyna et al.,(2011) reported 4/8 unrelated PWS carried at least one copy of p.Glu1200Lys variant in *GNPTAB* gene and established this as a founder mutation of the Asian population, originating from Pakistan and India.

Recurrence of this lysine variant in heterozygous condition (0.8%) segregating with affected status in our study favors the founder effect in Asians. Though the lysine variant is highly conserved across species (Consurf =9 (Glaser et al., 2003; Https://Consurf.Tau.Ac.Il, n.d.) with pathogenicity predictions and also *in silico* prediction of its effect on protein structure was shown to disrupt the helical segment which may be crucial for protein-protein interaction, its high frequency among South Asian ancestry (2.1%) in the gnomAD database is inconsistent with a causal role in stuttering pathology. Eight individuals in the south Asian population also had this homozygous variant indicating that this variant is not lethal, unlike *GNPTAB* homozygous variants observed in mucolipidosis. Hence this lysine variant is confirmed to be benign in the present study.

In a recent animal model study, 3- to 8-day old mice pups were engineered to carry two copies of the lysine mutation (Gnptab$^{mut/mut}$), resulting in significantly longer pauses in their spontaneous vocalizations consistent with some features of human stuttering. This was neither observed in littermates without the mutation (Gnptab$^{wt/wt}$) nor in heterozygous (Gnptab$^{mut/wt}$) littermates(Barnes, T. D., Wozniak, D. F., Gutierrez, J., Han, T. U., Drayna, D., & Holy, 2016). Based on this mouse model study, the causative role was well established for the homozygous lysine variant in the *GNPTAB* gene, while the heterozygous variant effect was notably similar to wild-type phenotypically. However, the significance of this variant acting in *trans* with other genetic determinants in other coding and non-coding exons could not be excluded. Further studies in this direction to identify new interacting genes or functionally related gene candidates in common pathways may clarify the causative role of this gene in stuttering.

In complex disorders, the genotype-phenotype correlation is rarely simple as dominance and recessive patterns for a given gene as described by Mendel. In many cases, multiple alleles contribute to a trait and include a variety of relationships between alleles (allelic interactions) that code for the same trait. Allelic dominance constantly depends on the relative influence of each allele responsible for the phenotype under given environmental conditions. Dominance and recessiveness are not essentially allelic properties but measured with respect to the effects of other alleles at the same locus. Additionally, dominance may change according to the level of organization of the phenotype and its variations highlight the complexity of understanding genetic influences on phenotypes (Miko, 2008). Two other *GNPTAB* homozygous mutations p.Ser321Gly and p.Ala455Ser engineered in mice, also displayed vocalization deficits traceable to abnormalities in astrocytes of corpus callosum (Han *et al.*, 2019).

STU 63 family with c.802A>C variant in *GNPTG* gene

This heterozygous variant was found only in the proband, but absent in other family members and hence it is confirmed to be *de novo*. It was not observed so far in the stuttering population but was reported in the gnomAD database in a heterozygous state with no information on MAF. In general, *de novo* variants are considered clinically significant due to constraints in natural selection and evolutionary conservation. The majority of genetic etiology studies of severe neurodevelopmental disorders associated with speech impairment were reported to be due to *de novo* mutations. They may be prime candidates when genetic diseases occur sporadically (Veltman, J. A., & Brunner, 2012). In our study, the role of this *de novo* variant in stuttering is ostensibly supported by a high conservation score. Investigation of the recurrence of this mutation is warranted in unrelated PWS that may provide further evidence of the *GNPTG* gene to neurobiological underpinnings of stuttering. Intriguingly, a recent study by Benito-Aragón *et al.*,(2020) had elucidated that *GNPTG* – a gene involved in the mannose-6-phosphate lysosomal targeting pathways – was significantly co-localized with the stuttering cortical network based on functional connectivity MRI and graph theory. This study had utilized a spatial similarity analysis approach that elucidated the topology of the stuttering cortical network by intersecting with genetic expression levels of previously reported genes for stuttering from the protein-coding transcriptome data of the Allen Human Brain Atlas.

Most of the mutations hitherto reported in stuttering are heterozygous. Hence a question arises: Are they dominant in stuttering in contrast to the recessive state observed in all mucolipidosis? Hence to study the impact of the *de novo* heterozygous missense variant identified in *GNPTG*, (i) quantification of mRNA by RT-PCR (ii) activity of lysosomal enzymes in plasma (iii) mucolipidosis screening was carried out between the affected and unaffected members of the family. Does this heterozygous condition have any impact on the expression and activity of the GNPTG enzyme? We also quantified two other genes *GNPTAB* and *NAGPA*, involved in mannose 6 phosphate formation to examine whether the defect in the *GNPTG* gene affects the expression of other components (Pohl *et al.*, 2009). Further *GNPTG* and *GNPTAB* genes encode different subunits of the same enzyme and there is a possible feedback regulation mechanism between them (Encarnação *et al.*, 2009).

If the variation affects the targeting function of the enzyme, it will not be targeted to lysosomes and hence will be secreted in the plasma. Thus the enzyme deficiency can be demonstrated by elevated lysosomal enzyme activity in plasma (Sheth *et al.*, 2012). Nevertheless, in our study the activity of GNPTG enzymes were not elevated, indicating that the enzyme might be successfully targeted to lysosomes. Also, the proband with stuttering did not have any symptoms of mucolipidosis and tested negative. We propose that, since the variation observed is in heterozygous condition, either the normal copy is sufficient or this variation does not affect the function of the enzyme. Similarly, there was no fold change in the mRNA level of the three genes between the affected (proband) and unaffected members (father, mother, and sister) of the family.

STU 34 family with c.131G>C variant in *NAGPA* gene

Only one isolated case of European descent has been reported to have this variant among the stuttering population studied (Raza et al., 2016). Observation of this variant in both affected and unaffected family members in our study suggests that this variant is less likely to have a causal effect. This may also be explained by incomplete penetrance that may fail to show any symptoms in some or could be due to phenocopies in affected members who may not be real carriers of variant but tend to display stuttering under environmental effects (Kang et al., 2010a). Also, variants observed in normal individuals may have caused stuttering but left un-informative owing to early recovery (Kazemi *et al.*, 2018); nevertheless, in the present study, we did not find any such recovery in this family.

Role of synonymous and noncoding variations

Overall, five synonymous variants and two noncoding variants were observed in our cohort. Synonymous mutations are often considered silent mutations due to \the degeneracy of genetic code. But they may have important consequences and are now recognized to be crucial in influencing gene expression, conformation, and cellular function (Sauna, Z. E., & Kimchi-Sarfaty, 2011). Complex disorders often tend to have multiple mutations. A mutation may not be detrimental individually but the joint effect of multiple variants in the same gene or different genes can contribute to a disorder but predictions are limited to a single variant (Liu, Watson, & Zhang, 2015).

Although our study has identified some of the reported variants, the perplexing question of causal role or the pathogenicity of a variant in the heterozygous state in stuttering or dysfluency disorder is still debatable. The process of speech-producing mechanism is believed to be highly heterogeneous due to its overlapping phenotypes with various genetic conditions and underlying etiology. Next generation sequencing based assays in individuals with stuttering will certainly throw light on complex disorders in terms of understanding the genetic heterogeneity, mutation burden in genes associated with speech-brain pathways.

5.2.3 EXOME SEQUENCING OF MULTIPLEX FAMILIES

The identification of genes with respect to complex disorders like stuttering, using linkage and GWAS studies are known to be time consuming and inconclusive respectively

(Kilpinen & Barrett, 2013). With the advent of NGS technology there is an increased interest to investigate the etiology of complex diseases to unravel the rare causative variants. Since these rare causal variants aggregate in families, family-based studies using NGS are more powerful. Hence multiplex families where one family with parent-offspring affected status and another family with affected sib pair were taken up for exome sequencing.

Status of already implicated genes and other potential mutations affecting the lysosomal function, in the two stuttering families

The status of the previously implicated genes *viz., GNPTAB, GNPTG, NAGPA* and *AP4E1* (Kang *et al.*, 2010; Raza *et al.*, 2015) in the affected stuttering individuals were verified in both the families. All the variants observed in the four genes were mostly intronic variants along with few missense that were synonymous and also nonsynonymous. But nonsynonymous variants were mostly benign except for a novel pathogenic missense variant (c.322G>A; p.Glu108Lys) in *NAGPA* gene in family STU 65 occurred in heterozygous condition.

In stuttering only four genes are implicated till date and is limited to only a single lysosomal pathway. This study has further investigated a list of 123 genes implicated in lysosomal function and did not identify any significant variation.

Further search for other putative pathways in the exome data

In STU 66 family, a segregation-based strategy was used to account for those gene variants overlapping with the affected members but absent in the unaffected members. Similarly, in STU 65 family, gene variants overlapping among the affected siblings were included. The possible candidate genes involved in both families were analyzed in two stages.

1. Separating out the **common genes among affected individuals in each family (276+294 genes) and comparing them** resulted in seven genes *(SLC36A1, C1orf167, SYNC, TM4SF1, MUC6, SPTBN5* and *MSRB1)* that were common to both the families with stuttering though they had different sets of variants in each gene. The identified genes have a role in signal transduction pathways especially at neuromuscular junctions.

Chapter 5 *Discussion*

2. From the common genes, **common coding variants among affected in each family** were sorted resulting in 31 gene variants (in 30 genes) in STU 66 family and 34 variants (in 34 genes) in STU 65 family. These genes were non overlapping between the two families. All the gene variants occurred in heterozygous condition except for *NLRP11* in STU 65 family that occurred as homozygous. Hence *NLRP11* gene could be a possible candidate gene in this family that shows consanguinity for three generations. Also the same family had a novel variant in previously implicated *NAGPA* gene. Since Stuttering is a complex disorder with extreme genetic heterogeneity identifying the high value target genes with variants in heterozygous condition is complicated. Hence all the 64 genes thus sorted, were subjected to two kinds on analysis.

  i. Exclusion of variants with heterozygous allele count >20 in GnomAD database that reduced the gene number from 64 to 35 (17 in STU 66 plus 18 in STU 65).

  ii. In another approach these 64 genes were subjected to pathway analysis to look for **common biological mechanisms**. Intriguingly, the list of genes that are possible candidate genes for stuttering among the two families are different, but fitting into common pathways. Among the 64 genes 41 were found to be involved in some or the other pathway. By carrying out an enrichment pathway analysis, 25 most relevant pathways encompassing 14 genes in two families were recognized (*COL4A2, COL6A3, COL6A6, ITGAX, LAMA5, ADAMTS9, CSGALNACT1, TMOD2, HTR2B, RSC1A1, TRPV2, WNK1, ARSD* and *SPTBN5*). On dissecting the functional discussion of these 14 genes, an interesting common link was identified. Most of the genes formed the **extra cellular matrix components and** are involved in **signaling** functions indicating an **overall cell communication deficit**.

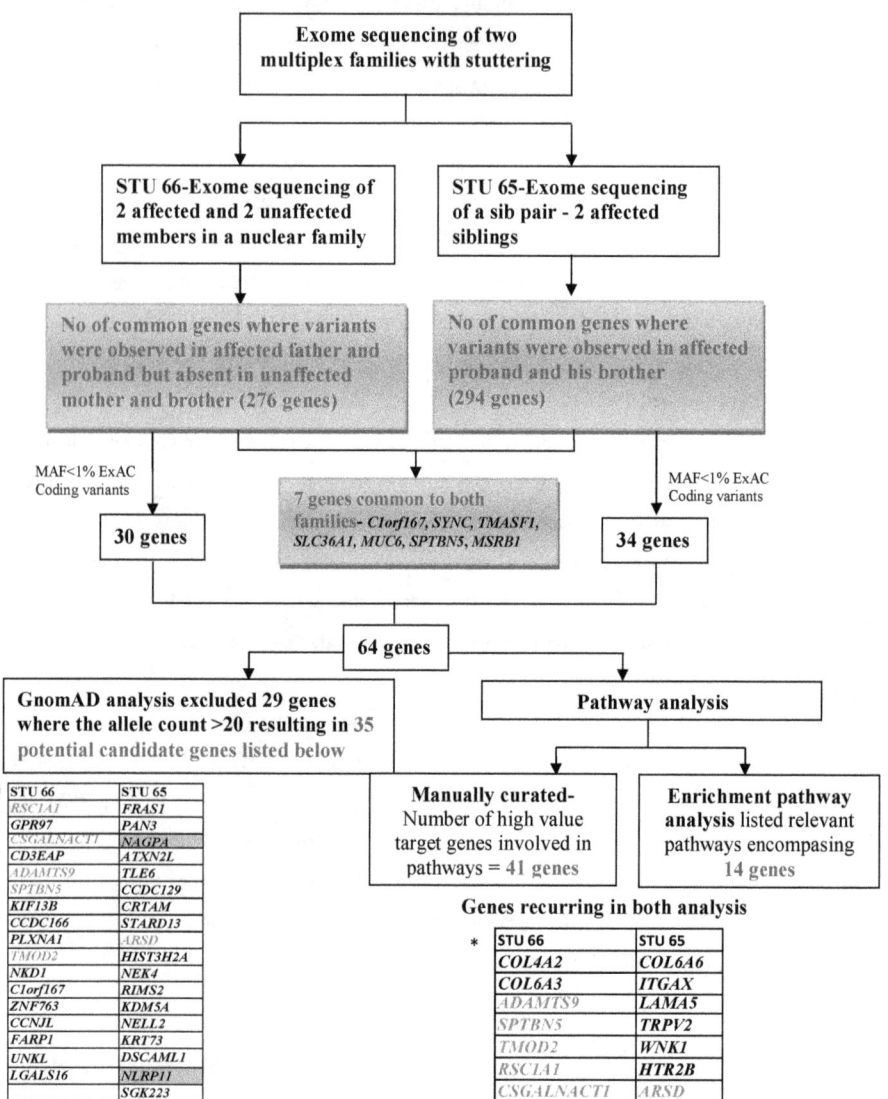

Figure 27: Flow chart depicting exome analysis of two multiplex stuttering families

Note: Genes that consistently occurred in different bioinformatic approaches are indicated in red. *NAGPA* gene implicated in published studies and *NLRP11* occurred in homozygous state in our study are highlighted

Figure 27 depicts the final list of potential candidate genes for stuttering, involved in **within-cell and cell-cell communication dynamics**. These genes encode for cytoskeletal proteins like intermediate filaments, ECM constituents (collagen, laminins, proteoglycans etc.), integrins that connect ECM to cytoskeletal proteins like actin, kinesin, etc., enzymes involved in ECM degradation, proteins involved in muscle contraction, proteins involved in vesicle transport, channels for transport of small molecules, receptors etc. Most of the genes that **consistently occurred** in the above analysis (*ADAMTS9, SPTBN5, TMOD2, RSCIA1, CSGALNACT1*) had novel variants.

ECM has three basic parts that involves basal lamina, interstitial matrix and perineuronal networks. ECM is dynamic, provides structural stability in the form of basement membrane, play role in signaling and are critical for neuroplasticity. (Hynes, 2009; Long & Huttner, 2019). Extracellular matrix provides an appropriate environment for the development and function of cells like **muscle cells and nerve cells** (Barros & Franco, 2011; Grzelkowska-Kowalczyk, 2016). In the present study, mutations in genes encoding collagen, laminins form part of the basement membrane, proteoglycans form the perineuronal nets all of which are important in neuroplasticity and maintaining synapses.

Cytoskeleton involves assembly of microfilaments, intermediate filaments and microtubule networks throughout the cell and besides their structural role are involved in signal transduction (Forgacs *et al.*, 2004; Sanghvi-Shah & Weber, 2017). Mutations in these genes may disrupt signaling.

Mutations in *TMOD2* and *SYNC* genes may disrupt muscle contraction. At neuro muscular junctions (NMJ), motor neurons release neurotransmitters that bind to post-synaptic receptors leading to contraction of muscles (Wu *et al.*, 2010). Hence disturbances in signaling system might occur at the neuromuscular junction that may influence speech disruption.

Thus, the genes identified were those involved in within and between cell communication and transport pathways indicating that the major disturbances in stuttering might be due to **disturbances in communication**. These pathways very well coincides with findings of neuroimaging (deficits in white matter tracts) (Chang *et al.*, 2015; Kronfeld-

Duenias *et al.*, 2018) and genetic animal studies (deficits in corpus callosum) (Han *et al.*, 2019) which concludes cell communication deficits as the major cause for stuttering. Also in a previous linkage study (Shugart *et al.*, 2004) that implicated chromosome 18, interesting candidate genes in desmoglein/desmocolin family and neuronal cadherin 2 gene that helps in cell-cell communication and cell adhesion was suggested. Such communications are found to be important in the neurons involved in the production of speech. In 19th century the traditional thinking was that the origin of speech and language could be localized to one part of our brain. However today neural bases are in fact found in the circuits that connect different regions of brain (Lieberman & Mccarthy, 2007).

In future, performing gene burden test to check for enrichment of variants in cases and controls would bring clarity on the genes involved in stuttering.

Using ES approach in highly multiplex stuttering families in this study led to interesting potential candidate genes involved in **signaling and transport**. A similar approach but in a more elaborate GWAS study, 10 potential candidate genes with significant p-values were identified to be strongly associated with stuttering (Kraft, 2010). However, we are aware that the present investigation is of a descriptive type and so the potential candidate genes identified should be viewed with caution because some of the variants may have no direct role in the development of the disorder. Yet, our results fit with the fact that stuttering is a multifactorial disease with a complex genetic background and hypothesize multiple and combined mechanisms involved in the genesis of stuttering.

The **variable expressivity of the disorder** could be explained by a strong genetic heterogeneity. ES in additional members would further narrow down on the variants involved and also functional studies of the identified variants would help in understanding the biological mechanism of stuttering or speech as such. The genes implicated in stuttering till date appear to be dominant as affected individuals had only one mutant copy (heterozygous condition). It appears to be associated with reduced level of functional protein (haploinsufficiency) in brain (rather than total absence).

Adding to the complexity exome sequencing addresses only coding regions. The remaining non coding regions that was initially considered as junk, 80% is now supposed to be biologically active of which 20% make functional RNAs that are involved in regulation (http://jonlieffmd.com/blog/extra-cellular-matrix-is-critical-to-neuroplasticity). The regulatory regions are 20 times bigger than protein coding regions. Thus, the complexity lies not only in the number of genes involved but in the amount of regulation of the genes.

CHAPTER 6

SUMMARY AND CONCLUSION

Persistent developmental stuttering is a complex speech disorder that disrupts the fluent speech in about 1% of population. It arises typically in childhood during the development of speech and language skills and most of the them recover spontaneously. Males are preferentially affected than females. Genetic basis of the disorder has steadily accumulated and has led to the identification of the genes *viz., GNPTAB, GNPTG* and *NAGPA* that play role in lysosomal targeting pathway.

Our study is the first targeted approach to scrutinize the **prevalence** of stuttering in India by screening school children. We collected epidemiological data on **risk factors** involved with emphasis on the impact of consanguinity and performed pedigree analysis to determine the **genetic basis** of the disorder.

In India no genetic studies on stuttering have been published till date and hence we initiated molecular genetics study from the database built by recruiting probands from schools and hospitals. Initially the molecular investigation involved the screening of the implicated **biological candidate genes *viz., GNPTAB, GNPTG* and *NAGPA*** among stuttering individuals was carried out. As a cost-effective strategy to screen all the three genes, we focused on the recurrence of the previously reported mutations in our study cohort of 64 probands. Further we used **exome sequencing** which is a powerful tool to elucidate genetic variants underlying stuttering in two highly multiplex families. The significant findings of the present study are recapitulated below:

- Screening 74,544 school children in the age group 2.5–16 years resulted in a **prevalence** of **0.46%** stuttering (N=342 children with stuttering) (95% CI=0.41% - 0.51%).
- A total of **380** probands were recruited from **schools and hospitals** with detailed information on important risk factors for stuttering that included: pre- and perinatal life; type of dysfluency; physical and emotional stress; handedness; the nature and age at onset of stuttering; parental marriage type, i.e. consanguinity; family history;

Chapter 6 *Summary and Conclusion*

family attitudes, including information on how they coped with the stuttering in daily life, their awareness of management/treatment; and personal reactions, e.g. anxiety, shyness.

- To avoid ascertainment bias, the two groups were subjected to statistical analysis separately.
- Pedigree analysis of **school data** showed that **familial incidence of stuttering (11%)** is higher than the general population incidence (1%) supporting the genetic nature of stuttering.
- On assessing the **risk factors associated with severity, sex** was significantly associated with severity, with female probands more likely to have a mild form of the disorder. A moderate effect was observed for increased severity with older **age of onset**. **Family history and consanguinity** within the pedigrees of probands were **not associated** with the severity of stuttering.
- **Familial aggregation** was examined using the **genealogical index of families (GIF), kinship group** and **probability of familial clustering (PFC)** tests as implemented in the R package FamAgg.
- The clustering of stuttering individuals was present in the analyzed pedigrees, especially within consanguineous families. As expected, the kinship group test identified large proportions of closely related affected individuals in consanguineous families. The sibling recurrence risk is high for consanguineous families and differs significantly from non-consanguineous counterparts. These tests provide evidence of the genetic nature of the disorder, indicating that a rare gene variant may be responsible for its expression.
- Comparing the school and hospital data a similar trend was observed among sex ratio, age at onset, birth order and sibship size.
- **Familial incidence** in school data (11%) is slightly higher than that of **hospital data (9%)**. Familial aggregation of affected relatives was also higher in school than hospital data. Further the difference observed in the familial aggregation in our two cohorts may be due to the difference in the ascertainment adopted. In the former it is a simple proband sampling from the general school population and in the latter it is physician referral from a speech therapy clinic.

Chapter 6 *Summary and Conclusion*

- **The genetic basis of the trait in our population was spotted by high familial incidence, familial aggregation and the sibling recurrence risk ratio.** Familial aggregation was high among consanguineous families although consanguinity did not seem to play a role in severity.
- A total of 64 unrelated probands with non-syndromic persistent stuttering were randomly selected from the database for mutational analysis. As a cost-effective strategy to screen all the three genes we focused on the recurrence of the previously reported mutations (9, 11, 13, 19 of *GNPTAB*; 1, 2, 9 &10 of *GNPTG* and 2, 6&7, 10 of *NAGPA)* in our study.
- Among these 64 probands screened, a total of **12 variants** were identified, which included **five nonsynonymous missense, five synonymous** and **two noncoding variants**. The variants found in the noncoding region (one in 5'UTR and another in intron) did not involve splice sites.
- Three unrelated probands harbored heterozygous missense variants at conserved coding positions across species [1,2] (p. Glu1200Lys in *GNPTAB*, p. Ile268Leu in *GNPTG* and p. Arg44Pro in *NAGPA*). Of these only one variant (p. Glu1200Lys in *GNPTAB*) co-segregated with the affected status while p. Ile268Leu in *GNPTG* gene was found to be a rare *de novo* variant.
-
- Most of the mutations so far reported in stuttering literature are by and large heterozygous, similar to that observed in our study. We wanted to comprehend how heterozygous mutations are involved in stuttering. Hence to study the **impact of** the *de novo* **heterozygous missense variation (c.802A>C; Ile268Leu)** identified in *GNPTG* gene, (i) at the level of mRNA expression and (ii) its effects on targeting function, quantification of mRNA by RT-PCR and activity of lysosomal enzymes in plasma by lysosomal enzyme study respectively was carried out in this family. We sought to observe if there are any differences in the expression of targeting genes and also targeting function of the lysosomal enzymes between the affected and unaffected members.
- Nevertheless, in our study the **activity of lysosomal enzymes were not elevated in plasma,** indicating that the enzyme might be successfully targeted to lysosomes.

- We propose that, since the variation observed is in heterozygous condition, either the normal copy is sufficient or this variation does not affect the function of the enzyme. Similarly, there was **no fold change in the mRNA level** of the three genes between the affected (proband) and unaffected members (father, mother and sister) of the family. Hence it was difficult to conclusively demonstrate the pathogenicity of this *de novo* mutation in stuttering.
- Although this study identified some previously reported variants that have been claimed to have a role in stuttering, we confirmed only one of these to be a likely causal *de novo* variant (p. Ile268Leu) in the *GNPTG* gene at an allele frequency of 0.8% (1/128) in the families with stuttering.
- In order to further explore the role of other genes involved in causing stuttering, we performed **exome sequencing in six individuals** from two multiplex families. One family with **parent-offspring** affected status and another family with affected **sib pair** was taken up.
- The **status of the previously implicated genes** *viz., GNPTAB, GNPTG, NAGPA, AP4E1* (Kang *et al.*, 2010; Raza *et al.*, 2015) in affected stuttering individuals were verified in both the families. All the variations observed in the four genes were mostly intronic variations along with few missense variants that were synonymous and nonsynonymous. These nonsynonymous variations were benign variations except for a heterozygous novel missense variant **(c.322G>A, p. Glu108Lys) in *NAGPA* gene**, that was predicted as pathogenic by *in silico* methods, in the sib pair of family STU 65.
- Exome sequencing analysis of two multiplex families with stuttering, firstly identified seven genes *(SLC36A1, C1orf167, SYNC, TM4SF1, MUC6, SPTBN5* and *MSRB1)* segregating with the affected, that were common to both the families though they had different sets of variants in each gene. These genes with variants seem to collectively play role in **signal transduction pathways** that might disrupt signaling between neurons or at neuromuscular junction.
- Secondly **common coding variants** segregating with the affected members in each family (31 variants spread across **30 genes** in STU 66 family and 34 variants in **34 genes** in STU 65 family), were further analyzed.

Chapter 6 — Summary and Conclusion

  I. Exclusion of variants that had heterozygous allele count >20 in GnomAD database reduced the gene number from 64 to **35** (17 in STU 66 and 18 in STU 65).
  II. High value target genes was sorted by looking for **common biological mechanisms** and **enrichment pathway analysis. Fourteen tentative candidate genes** enriching the putative pathways were identified that form the **extra cellular matrix (ECM) components and those involved in signaling and transport.** Most of the remaining genes were indicated as interactors.

- From the analysis above certain genes were **consistently observed as potential candidate genes that are involved in within-cell and cell-cell communication.** The pathways arrived in our study very well coincide with the findings of deficits in white matter tracts and corpus callosum, which point to the cell communication deficits as the major cause for stuttering that is also reported in literature.

- **Limitations of the work** include recruitment of children from only two areas of Tamil Nadu (Chennai and Salem) for the genetic epidemiology study. By combining the data from Chennai and Salem it was assumed that there were no differences between the two populations that might influence stuttering. Referral by class teachers might have contributed to a slight underestimate in stuttering prevalence. Although the sibling recurrence risk ratio was higher within consanguineous than non-consanguineous families, the additional risk was minimal in general terms, given the heterogeneity of this complex disorder.

- While screening for biologically implicated genes for stuttering, we limited the screening to only previously reported exons, to increase the chance of its recurrence with respect to our population. In the event of screening all the exons in the three genes, more variants (including compound heterozygotes) may be added to the list.

- A synonymous variant c. 1485C>T in *NAGPA* gene (predicted as benign) occurred in homozygous condition in 42 stuttering individuals but in heterozygous condition in the presence of another missense variant c.1394 C>T (predicted to be benign) in the same gene in 22 stuttering individuals. The significance of its excessive occurrence was not addressed at this time of study but in future, segregation of this missense variant in the 22 proband's nuclear families, could verify its role in stuttering. In the exome sequencing performed in two families, all the affected and unaffected individuals were homozygous for c.1485C>T synonymous variant with absence of the missense variant c.1394 C>T.

- In the exome sequencing performed in the present investigation, the **putative pathways identified are of descriptive type** and so the potential candidate genes identified should be viewed with caution because some of the variants may have no direct role in the development of the disorder. Yet, our results fit with the fact that **stuttering is a multifactorial disease with a complex genetic background** and hypothesize multiple and combined mechanisms involved in the genesis of stuttering.

- ES in additional members would further narrow down the variants involved and also functional studies of the identified variants would help in understanding the biological mechanism of stuttering or speech as such.

- Overall, this study enabled the investigator to **develop a stuttering database** that includes multiplex families, which could be taken up for further investigations. Better understanding of the underlying biological mechanism of stuttering would help us to develop therapies and early intervention.

- Epidemiological studies help in establishing the burden of disease and also in identifying its risk factors. Based on this some of the funds for education development programs can be allocated while planning to screen for speech related difficulties. Although the prevalence of stuttering observed in Tamil Nadu (0.46%) indicates its relatively low occurrence in the overall community an exercise as suggested above will help to identify other speech disorders also for early intervention not only in the form of therapy but also in setting up awareness campaigns, self-help groups at various levels. Without appropriate education, parents tend to blame the child for being dysfluent on purpose. Hence counseling can be directed to both the parent and child. In societal level such efforts can change the manner in which the disability is perceived.

CPSIA information can be obtained
at www.ICGtesting.com
Printed in the USA
BVHW051329280423
663226BV00011B/1007